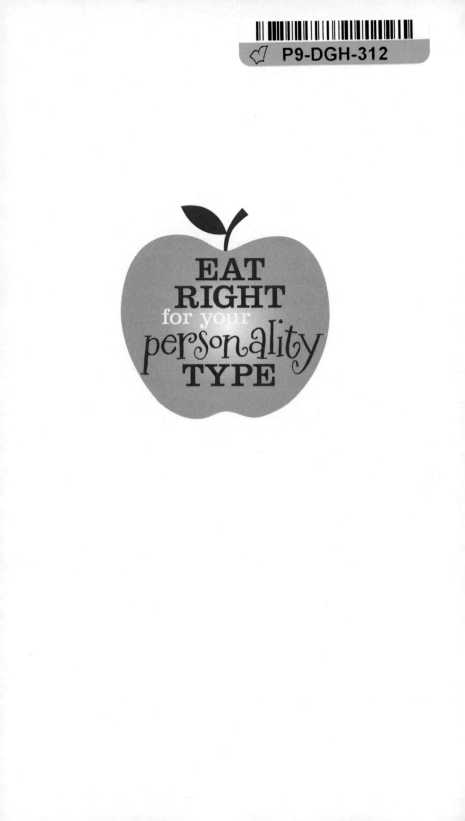

EAT RIGHT
for your
personality
TYPE

EAT RIGHT for your personality TYPE

How to Work with YOUR Personality to Create the Perfect Diet for You

KAREN KNOWLER

HAY HOUSE

HAY HOUSE
Australia • Canada • Hong Kong • India
South Africa • United Kingdom • United States

First published and distributed in the United Kingdom by:
Hay House UK Ltd, 292B Kensal Rd, London W10 5BE
Tel: (44) 20 8962 1230; Fax: (44) 20 8962 1239
www.hayhouse.co.uk

Published and distributed in Australia by:
Hay House Australia Ltd, 18/36 Ralph St, Alexandria NSW 2015
Tel: (61) 2 9669 4299; Fax: (61) 2 9669 4144
www.hayhouse.com.au

Published and distributed in the Republic of South Africa by:
Hay House SA (Pty), Ltd, PO Box 990, Witkoppen 2068
Tel/Fax: (27) 11 467 8904
www.hayhouse.co.za

Published and distributed in India by:
Hay House Publishers India, Muskaan Complex, Plot No.3, B-2,
Vasant Kunj, New Delhi – 110 070
Tel: (91) 11 4176 1620; Fax: (91) 11 4176 1630
www.hayhouse.co.in

Distributed in Canada by:
Raincoast, 9050 Shaughnessy St, Vancouver, BC V6P 6E5
Tel: (1) 604 323 7100; Fax: (1) 604 323 2600

A catalogue record for this book is available from the British Library.

ISBN: 978-1-84850-577-3

Printed and bound in Great Britain by TJ International, Padstow, Cornwall.

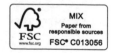

this book is dedicated to you
x

Contents

Acknowledgements

Thank you to family, friends, colleagues and clients who have shared so much of themselves with me that I could uncover this powerful work.

Thank you to Ali's Diamonds 2009, whose support and encouragement provided the resounding 'YES' for getting this book out into the world.

Thank you to Julia McCutchen who assisted me in pulling my ideas together in a way that worked.

Thank you to BG for your unwavering support, patience and tenaciousness.

Thank you to all at Hay House for your belief in this work and helping me to spread the word.

Thank you to Katie Foster and the rest of my fabulous team for all of your invaluable back-at-the-ranch support, which enables me to do what I do.

Thank you to Kendall SummerHawk, Ali Brown and Fabienne Fredrickson who have impacted me, my work and my world more than you will ever know. I am forever grateful.

Thank you to Tony for all your support every step of the way; this work has been made all the deeper and richer for everything you've shared with me.

Thank you, Luke, for letting Mummy write and being all that you are. I am so proud of you.

Preface

There are people all around the world right now who are eating something and feeling bad about it.

It might be because they know it's not a healthy thing to eat, or because they know it will make them gain weight, that it will exacerbate a health condition or sensitivity, that its source is not ethical or sustainable, that they're eating something they don't enjoy, or maybe they even had to steal it because they didn't have the money to buy it.

Perhaps you also have had times like this where you ate something and didn't feel good about it? If you're like 80 per cent+ of the Western population, this might even be the story of your life.

How would it be if you could find a way of eating that nourished you on every level, that was comprised of foods that were a perfect fit for you in every way, that made you look and feel the way you want to look and feel, and that you knew that, *no matter what you ate*, you would always be able to feel at peace with, while the majority of the time you would easily and naturally make choices that felt 100 per cent great to you?

If this sounds like an impossible dream, then I'm here to wake you up from your slumber.

Your first step to food freedom begins with understanding the single biggest factor in your eating and dietary patterns – the one thing which, more than anything else, has created your food story, your body, your health, your eating habits and your energy levels.

That one defining factor is something totally within your control. You've carried it about with you from the day you were born. You won't find it in a bottle, jar or diet book. It's not something you've learned, experienced or heard about from your neighbour.

It's not your blood type, your metabolic type or which part of the world you were born in, nor the first food you ever tasted.

No, the single biggest factor in your joy and your pain around food is closer than you think, so close in fact that you couldn't even see it – until now...

Introduction

It took me over a decade to figure it out.

After coaching and speaking globally with thousands of men and women about their eating habits, it finally hit me:

There are different types of eater.

Specifically, I'm talking eating 'styles' or 'personalities', if you will. The part of you that you might call 'you' but really has simply become your *modus operandi* because of a whole host of contributing factors which have shaped the food choices that you make today.

Each of these different types has individual ways of thinking, feeling and acting around food, for a whole host of varied reasons – reasons which may not always serve our best interests and that often bring as much pain as they do pleasure.

Pretty fascinating, I'm sure you'll agree.

Allow me to explain.

Imagine that you are sitting in a restaurant and you witness a party of 10 diners take their seats and pick up a copy of the menu.

If you could mind-read and were to listen in on the thoughts of each diner in turn, you would be quite amazed at the diversity of inner monologues going on.

What you would hear as you moved around the table would be something like this: 'I'm going to get the pasta and not have dessert because I want to be out of here as soon as possible.' 'I'm going to go for the fish in white wine sauce with fresh garlic potatoes and crusty bread and have the chocolate torte for dessert… because I'm feeling really naughty!' 'Now, which of these looks like the healthiest meal on the menu?' 'I've totally had enough today. I'm going to eat whatever I want and get drunk to boot – yeah!' 'Hmmm… what can I see on here that's carb-free and has fewer than 500 calories?' 'Which of these do I most fancy today?' 'OK, now, where are the vegan options?' 'What haven't I eaten before? I'm going to have THAT!' 'I don't know what on Earth to choose… Ugh.' 'What's great for sharing? Who's going to share with me?' Any of these sound familiar? Perhaps you hear yourself, or some version of you, somewhere in there?

By 'eavesdropping' on this fun and diverse group, you've just been introduced to the 10 different types of eater:

1. The Functional Eater

2. The Sensual Eater

3. The Intellectual Eater

4. The Emotional Eater

5. The Focused Eater

6. The Intuitive Eater

7. The Conscious Eater

8. The Experimental Eater

9. The Confused Eater

10. The Social Eater

Over the next few pages you are going to learn something really fascinating about yourself. You're going to discover what type of eater YOU are.

It might be something you already feel you have a handle on, having learned a little about each type just now – maybe merely seeing the names listed above has got you thinking, or, just as possible… what you are about to discover might be incredibly enlightening to you.

Either way, by learning your current type, or combination of types (rare is the person who is 100 per cent one type, by the way), you will be in a position to:

- Decide if your eating style is really the best fit for you.

- Decide how you want to move forward with your type/s, or whether you want to swap, release or completely change the way you approach eating.

- Decide what experience/results with food you want to have next, and why.

- Decide which foods you are going to play with to make that happen.

The truth is, right now your 'default' style, even though it is likely to be largely unconscious, has been working for you on some level and has been yielding payoffs – which is why you're still using it – but it is also very possibly presenting challenges to you as well. By learning more about each type you will be in the wonderful position where you can take a step back from what has gone before and handpick the type, or combination of types, that is going to be the best fit for what you want for your body, health and lifestyle. This will enable you to rewrite your unique 'food story' with clarity, intention and a definite sense of purpose rather than letting randomness rule, or even *ruin*, your life.

As you will see, there's no end to what you can create!

A Recipe for Success

Through the two life-changing parts of this book – The 10 Types and The 10 Possibilities – I'm going to walk you step-by-step through the process that will change the way you see and experience yourself, and food, forever.

As someone who has gone from one end of the spectrum to the other (junk-food eater and butcher-shop worker to raw food eater, coach and teacher), I can personally vouch for the power of making informed and thoughtful choices around food. As I learned to acknowledge the Conscious, Intuitive and Intellectual Eaters in me, my whole body, health and energy levels changed, and soon after my whole life with it!

Even today I am still playing with the different styles and combinations possible to create new experiences and learn new things about myself and my body in every new chapter of my life. By experimenting and having fun you will learn really quickly what 'recipe for success' works best for you, and in the meantime you get to enjoy every step of the journey.

By the way, in case you were wondering if I'm going to tell you *what* to eat, the answer is an unequivocal 'No!' As someone who has tried diets (and failed miserably) in the past, I finally came to understand why most people struggle: the fact is, only the Intellectual, Focused and Confused Eaters actually like being told what to eat! The rest of us resent it or resist it with a passion. So with this in mind, and because I want you to own your individual choices completely, whatever they may be, I'm not going to tell you one thing about what to eat. I'm simply going to lay out the life-changing options before you. Yes, you can eat cake all day if that's what you really, *really* want…

Having said that, just so you know, I definitely fly the flag for optimum well-being. We have all been given an amazing body that is incredibly powerful and tolerant and capable of far more than we will ever know. The thought of that and of exploring those possibilities really excites me, hence why my own personal journey took me into the world of raw food (for maximum nutrition, life-force energy, weight maintenance and a peaceful relationship with food).

The Power of Choice

Never underestimate the power of what you put into your body. Through my work I have come to see time and time again that what you put into your mouth often has a much bigger impact on your life than what you allow to come out of it. The quality of your cells is dependent on the quality of food you put into YOU. From that comes the quality of your health, your energy, your skin, your eyesight, your hair… the list goes on. And as you will see for yourself, if and when you start to do things differently, the food you eat will also have a huge impact on the way you think, the way you feel and the relationship you have with yourself, your body and the world around you. In short, what you eat can change *everything*.

For a very long time as a species we had to eat whatever was available. Now we have the power to choose. What has not been discussed until now is the multitude of choices that truly are possible.

When you combine knowledge of the different eating styles with the many health and life experiences possible, you will be amazed at what new doors can and will be blown wide open to you.

If this sounds like something you would like to know more about, then you are in for an extraordinary ride!

Welcome to the plate of possibilities. I look forward to helping you move from curiosity to clarity, and to helping you create the most delicious and satisfying possibilities for YOU.

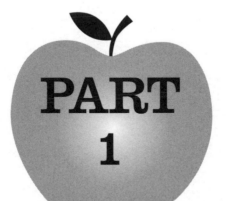

PART 1

the 10 types

CHAPTER 1
What Type of Eater Are You?

Discovering what type of eater you are will change everything for you.

Having been a food coach since 1999, I still marvel at how many years it took me to become aware of how distinctly different people are around their approach to food and eating, and then to categorize those behaviours into the 10 'types' that genuinely cover all the bases. Once I finally uncovered the 10 types and started to share this information with others, they, too – without exception – had an 'Aha!' moment, as in *why on Earth didn't I recognize this before?*

My thoughts on this are that generally we are all so busy being busy that we simply don't have time to ask questions or think too much about our relationship to food. Instead, we just mentally categorize someone as a 'fussy' eater, or a 'calorie-obsessed' eater or an 'I can give him anything and he'll eat it' kind of eater. But dig a little deeper and you'll find that you, just like everyone else, have an eating 'personality' comprised of one or more Eater Types, and that this personality dictates *everything* that you think, feel and do around food. *How's that for fascinating?*

To be clear, even though all 10 types are very different, there is no 'ideal type' for you to be – no right or wrong, as such – although there is a hierarchy of sorts, and definitely a 'ladder' of evolution when it comes to eating. So if you're the type of person who really likes to explore the deeper layers of things, or if you're just generally curious about how the different types play into one another, then you'll want to check that out at the back of the book (page 249).

If you're not so concerned about the details, though, and simply want to eat and enjoy what you're eating, then you'll be pleased to know that there is a type or combination of types that will best suit you and your desires, goals and circumstances. And the good news is – you get to choose!

Yes, that's right, no matter who you are or where you've been on your food journey to date, you get to *choose* your future experience. Because what I have also learned is that, while all of us have a 'default setting', it *can* be changed – but not until you:

- know what type/s you are now
- know what you want your next experience regarding food to be (e.g. weight loss, more energy, increased nutrition, becoming a 'foodie', etc.)

Once you know this, you're in a position to weigh up which Eater Type profile would best enable you to have that particular experience and/or gain specific benefits and results.

Drawing on my own and others' experiences, I can say for sure that when you have this clarity about yourself and what you truly desire for yourself, then changing your type can actually happen in a heartbeat.

You see, I truly believe that inside each and every one of us, all 10 types reside. You have just chosen to 'channel' one or more of them right now due to a range of factors unique to you, all of which are largely unconscious and have been encouraged by your upbringing and environment. However, the good news is that if your type is no longer working for you, or if you want to experience something different, then you can evolve, trade or reconfigure which type/s you move forward with very easily.

Conscious Eating

The benefits of choosing your type are many. Aside from getting the experience that you want (you'll learn about your various options in Chapter 4), becoming more conscious about food is always a good thing. Sadly, many of the people feeling lousy right now are doing so because they *aren't* conscious about what they put into their bodies. We've come way too far now to pretend that we don't know that what we eat has the power to make or break our health. Our healthcare system is stretched to the limit by people requiring long-term care or emergency intervention for diet-related illnesses such as strokes, heart disease, diabetes and morbid obesity. It's time to take responsibility for your own health before you end up somewhere that you don't want to be. This book will show you how.

But don't worry: taking responsibility doesn't have to be dull, boring or anything like hard work. Far from it. By discovering your default type/s, choosing your desired experience, and then experimenting with the different types within you, you will *automatically* be taking responsibility for what you eat – except this time, as you move towards the relationship that you *really* want with food and the personal reality that you want to create with it, it will feel like the most exciting journey on Earth!

Your Own Personal Coach

In the pages that follow I'm going to be your personal Eat Right For Your Personality Type (ERFYPT) coach. I'm totally committed to helping you discover this fascinating information about yourself and helping you to set yourself free – just like I discovered for myself in the mid-1990s.

To get us started, together we're going to find out two very important things about you:

1. What your current relationship with food and eating is like, and how happy (or not) you are with it.

2. What your current 'Eater Type' profile is, and specifically how that's been serving you (or not).

Once we have this information, I'm going to share with you detailed information about each of the 10 types, so you can read up more about your own personal type/s and get clearer on how they have – or haven't – been working for you.

And, of course, if you want to (and this is just as fun!) you can then put your newfound knowledge towards helping your friends and family to learn more about themselves and *their* Eater Types.

So, are you ready to begin your life-changing journey to clarity, insight and freedom?

If you are, then it all starts here…

Where Am I Now?

Get a piece of paper, or a notebook, and a pen or pencil.

Now think: on a scale of 1–10, with 10 being 'delighted' and 1 being 'seriously depressed', how happy do you currently feel about the way that you eat?

Write the number down.

How do you feel about that score? Write your answer down.

If your score is under 10, what do you see as the biggest problem that prevents your score from being a 10? Write your answer down.

Ultimate Eater Quiz

Answer the following questions on a scale of 1–5, with 1 being 'not at all', 3 being 'sometimes' and 5 being 'all the time':

1. My eating routine suits the amount of time, money and effort I am prepared to put into it.

2. In my home, I can make or find delicious foods quickly if I need to.

3. I love everything that I eat.

4. I gain pleasure from my food.

5. From a nutritional standpoint, I am happy with the food choices that I make.

6. I know exactly what goes into my food and am happy and confident about what I am eating.

7. I only eat for hunger-related reasons.

8. I purchase food for reasons other than emotion-led ones.

9. I know exactly what kind of body, level of health and energy I am looking to create.

10. I have a plan to get me to where I want to go with my food/dietary journey.

11. I tune in to my body to know what foods are good for me.

12. I only eat foods that I know really work well for me.

13. I feel ethically and morally happy about the food choices that I make.

14. I take time to source and buy myself the best foods that I can.

15. I try new foods at least once a month.

16. My diet is varied and diverse.

17. If I don't know if something's good for me, I find out.

18. I proactively educate myself about food and nutrition.

19. I enjoy food with friends as often as feels good to me.

20. I have found a way of eating in company that feels comfortable to me.

Now add up your total score, tallying up across all 20 questions.

Your score will be out of a possible 100.

Write down your score.

What Your Score Says about You

What does your score tell you about your current way of eating? Do you notice any themes in your answers? Have you learned anything new about yourself?

Take a few moments to jot down your response to what you've just learned.

What we just did here via the Ultimate Eater Quiz is see where your strengths and weaknesses are in relation to each of the 10 types. Rare, if not unheard of, is the person who scores a 5 on every question. To do so you probably would have spent years, if not decades, paying close attention to yourself and your diet, *and* the life, health and body that you want to create. It's entirely possible to score a full 100, but my guess is, if you're reading this book, you probably still have some way to go!

Please know that every moment that you spend contemplating your diet will be a moment that will pay you back handsomely for the rest of your life. By working your way through this book (and, by the way, by the time you've completed this first chapter, half the 'work' will be done), you will have done more for yourself and your future than you can possibly imagine.

So, by this point you know:

• How happy you currently feel about your food and eating.

- What you think is the biggest problem preventing you from experiencing optimum joy around food and eating.

- Where your strengths and weaknesses lie in relation to having a well-rounded, 'ultimate' relationship and experience with food.

- If there are any particular themes or patterns regarding your strengths and weaknesses around food.

Now that you have this invaluable information under your belt, it's time to do THE QUIZ – the one you've been waiting for.

It's time to find out what your current Eater Type profile is. I can't wait to help you find out!

The What Type of Eater Are YOU? Quiz

For each of the following five statements, please read through each of the 10 possible answers and then select the ONE (and only one) that *best fits* how you are around food today.

1. In my normal day-to-day life I...

A. eat to feel full or satisfied, rarely eating when not hungry.

B. love to eat – it doesn't matter what it is so long as I love it!

C. decide what is most appropriate for my nutritional or calorific needs and then eat accordingly.

D. eat whether I am hungry or not, and sometimes not even food I actually enjoy.

E. think about what my current life and body goals are and eat according to what I am trying to achieve.

F. tune in to my body and ask what food or drink would be the most appropriate for it right now.

G. choose foods that are in line with my ethics, morals and principles – those come first.

H.   eat whatever is around, and hope there's something new and exotic in the fridge that will get me excited.

I.   usually don't know what to eat. My food choices vary depending on many different factors, and it depends on where I am in my learning at the time.

J.   eat what other people are eating, unless I really don't like it.

2. If I could eat just one thing it would be...

A.   it honestly doesn't matter as long as it fills me up!

B.   a piece of chocolate (or a whole bar!) or something really decadent that I love.

C.   my favourite superfood of the moment.

D.   whatever I feel like at the time, and I don't have to be hungry.

E.   something that keeps me mean and lean!

F.   I cannot tell you; it's whatever is right in this moment, and that changes all the time.

G.   something local, organically grown and made with love.

H.   pretty much anything, so long as it tastes good or looks interesting.

I.   I honestly have no clue!

J.   what someone else has made me, hopefully!

3. The thing that I love most about food and eating is...

A.   waiting for true hunger and then refuelling with just enough to feel satiated again.

B.   just about everything! I love food and I love the way it makes me feel.

C.   how what we eat can make or break our human experience.

D. oftentimes I don't love much about it; it is frequently the bane of my life.

E. it helps me get where I want to go.

F. how my body reacts to different foods in different ways, and what I can learn about myself as a result.

G. through the choices I make I get to make the world a better place.

H. there is so much variety out there! I love trying new things – variety is the spice of life!

I. when I get it right I enjoy it, but much of the time it is a minefield for me.

J. it's a way of bringing people together; life is so much richer for it.

4. What I don't much like about food and eating is...

A. it slows me down! Sometimes I don't want to have to stop and eat but I have to.

B. sometimes I feel a bit overindulged and not so great in my body.

C. the health professionals keep changing their information and advice. It drives me crazy.

D. I usually feel out of control with it and I really wish I didn't.

E. the world is not ideally set up to help me eat the way I want.

F. I can't always 'hit the spot' with what I'm eating or drinking, and feel that something's missing.

G. I believe that we should all be generally eating less than we are, so for me it is having to eat at all. I would much rather live on fresh air, pure water and sunshine.

H. there isn't enough time on the planet to explore all the wonderful foods that surround us!

I.   that I cannot find the right way for me. I don't know if I'm ever going to figure it out.

J.   it's not that exciting really, unless shared with good company.

5. The perfect foodie lifestyle for me would be...

A.   quick, easy and delicious – and even better if I don't have to make it!

B.   full of yummy foods that make me moan with pleasure!

C.   perfectly balanced nutritionally, giving my body everything that it needs.

D.   one that would feel comforting and have lots of treats in it.

E.   whatever gets me the results I am seeking and fits in with the life I am creating.

F.   having enough food in the fridge so I always have plenty to choose from, because I never know what I might fancy.

G.   peaceful, conscious and whole.

H.   incredibly varied, anything goes!

I.   100 per cent tailored to me, all mapped out and I know what I'm eating, when and why.

J.   living in a household or community where we come together to eat each day.

Results

Write down the different letters that you have chosen for the five statements. You might find that you have five letters all the same, or a combination of anything between two and five different ones, such as two Bs, one C, and two Fs. These reveal your Eater Type profile, as you can see from the table that follows.

The 10 Different Eater Types

The Functional Eater	Mostly As	see page **14**
The Sensual Eater	Mostly Bs	see page **24**
The Intellectual Eater	Mostly Cs	see page **36**
The Emotional Eater	Mostly Ds	see page **47**
The Focused Eater	Mostly Es	see page **58**
The Intuitive Eater	Mostly Fs	see page **69**
The Conscious Eater	Mostly Gs	see page **80**
The Experimental Eater	Mostly Hs	see page **92**
The Confused Eater	Mostly Is	see page **103**
The Social Eater	Mostly Js	see page **115**

On page 257 you will find a template for creating your own unique Eat Right For Your Personality Type Personal Success Blueprint. This blueprint will help you to keep a record of the most important information about your ERFYPT journey, so that you can get clear on exactly where you are now and what needs to happen to reach the magical score of 100 (if you want to) – *and* create your chosen eating and food-related experiences. For now, please go ahead and read about each of your current Eater Types on pages 14–124; once you've done that, have a look at the other Eater Types to familiarize yourself with those, too.

Once you've done that, continue on to Chapter 2, where I'll explain what to do with what you've learned so far.

Have fun!

THE FUNCTIONAL EATER 🍏

Functional Eaters don't dislike food or eating, but you could be forgiven for thinking that they do! It is not necessarily their priority that everything they eat is the best or the most delicious possible (although they'd rather it is, given the choice) – they're just not always that choosy! They simply want to eat and they want to eat *now*, so that they can get on with life and do what they consider to be more important things. For the Functional Eater, it is all about speed and convenience.

The Functional Eater's view –

- on food: 'Nice'
- on eating: 'Inconvenient'
- on self-catering: 'Ugh'
- on takeaways: 'Great'
- on being personally catered for: 'Heaven'
- on eating out: 'Yum!'
- on changing their diet: 'As long as it stays quick and easy, I'm open to it.'

The Functional Eater and Pleasure

Functional Eaters love it when…

- **food is quick and easy to prepare.** Functional Eaters love the microwave, the grill, the quick-cook rice, pasta or soups and, at the healthier end of the scale, the blender. (The healthier ones will shun the microwave but tend to resent having to chop, grate or do anything from scratch, seeing those five minutes as a massive inconvenience and more like five hours.)

- **they can have grab-and-go pre-prepared foods.** If they can grab their meal off a shelf or out of the fridge and be eating it in a minute or less, the Functional Eater is a very happy bunny.

- **they eat out at a restaurant.** What better than simply to order off a menu and have everything you want delivered straight to the table with no effort whatsoever? When the food happens to be a perfect fit for the Functional Eater on all levels, this is their idea of eating nirvana.

The Functional Eater's idea of heaven: 'A fridge full of delicious pre-prepared foods that I love or, even better, a personal chef to serve it up for me so I can grab it and go.'

The Functional Eater and Pain

Functional Eaters struggle when…

- **there's no ready-made food around.** Having to take the time to make something sends the Functional Eater into a spin of frustration. At times like this the quality of their diet will go massively downhill, leading to snacking on random things, not eating enough or simply not eating a well-balanced diet because they won't take the time to make it so.

- **they get bored of eating the same thing day after day.** This can easily happen because the Functional Eater will happily gravitate towards a routine for maximum efficiency, but when it doesn't taste good anymore, that's when they have to give some time and energy to reassessing and figuring something else out.

- **they change the way they do things.** If a Functional Eater decides to get healthy or eat according to more structured rules, this will automatically mean a new way of shopping, prepping and all manner of other considerations which they'd honestly rather not have to deal with. In fact, budget allowing, this would be when they would hire a personal chef or nutritionist rather than having to learn it all for themselves.

The Functional Eater's idea of hell: 'Having a fridge full of ingredients that I have to do something with.'

If This Is You

If you are a Functional Eater, or if this fits part of your Eater Type profile, bookmark this page for a second and turn to Chapter 2 (page 126), where there are three short (but revealing!) questions I'd like you to have a think about. These will help you get more in touch with how being a Functional Eater has worked for you *and* caused issues. You don't have to do anything with this information just yet, but don't skip it; it is vital. Take this opportunity to reflect on things; you may well have one or two 'Aha!' moments that could be of tremendous value to you. Once you've done that, come back to this page and keep reading.

· ·

Case Study: Dylan, 28, London

When Dylan and I first started working together, his main desire was to 'get healthy, lose some weight, gain more energy and learn more about what's good for me.'

As a typical Functional Eater, Dylan usually stuck to eating things he knew he liked, and he tended to eat and drink the same things on a daily basis. However, because he had never been interested in healthy eating before, his tendency was to go for high-sugar, high-fat foods that would taste good and fill him up – until he started to feel overweight, bloated and low in energy. Then he knew he had to change.

As Dylan's desires were clear and specific, we had some firm terrain upon which to build. It was clear to me that, for him to fulfil those desires, he was going to have to start embodying the habits and preferences of the Intellectual Eater and the Focused Eater. This would ensure that he became more aware of what he was eating, and that he ate according to the weight loss goal he was trying to reach. By default he would absolutely increase his energy levels as he lost the weight and increased the quality of his food.

Taking Dylan's 'Functional' nature into account, we began with very simple, easy to implement steps, including a shopping trip to help him learn which healthy foods would be quick and simple to prepare or eat, and that would help him reach his weight loss goal. This one step was pivotal for Dylan who, having left home at a relatively young age and having never been around friends or family who ate healthily, honestly did not have a clue where to start.

Once we had worked out a basic menu plan that required very little input on his part, he was well away! We focused on high-quality, high-nutrient and low-fat foods, while still building in some healthy treats. Dylan loved this, as the new plan required no more thinking or doing on his part than his previous diet, but he could quickly see and feel the difference.

Needless to say, within just a few short weeks Dylan had not only lost the excess 10 lb and gained a lot more energy, he was developing quite a passion for nutrition – so much so, he had even started considering training to be a nutritionist in his spare time.

· ·

The Benefits of Being a Functional Eater

- Uses food as fuel, rather than as entertainment or pleasure.

- Frees up more energy for other projects, outside of eating.

- Keeps food and eating as something separate to other aspects of your life.

- An approach to food and eating that is straightforward and simple.

- Helps with weight loss, choosing the right foods *and* not overeating at the same time.

Adopting the Habits of a Functional Eater

- Allow less time to prepare food and eat it than usual.

- Eat more simply.

- Decrease or eliminate the amount of fancy or 'seductive' foods you eat and buy.

- Allow someone else to make your food for you, without stressing about what it is.

- Keep reminding yourself that food should primarily be viewed as fuel and that there are more exciting things in life you can be creating or focusing on.

Integrating with Other Types

Integrated with the Sensual Eater

As the Sensual Eater is at the opposite end of the scale, this is a very fun and enjoyable mix. When this occurs, the Functional Eater gets to slow down, really enjoy food and see food as more than fuel – which they secretly enjoy! This is a joyful union when the Functional Eater is satisfied by delicious, simply prepared foods that are served to them beautifully presented with care and attention. When this happens they can take their time to enjoy all the insights that come to them as they expand their relationship with food and start to see it as something that can help them enjoy *life* more, and stop them scurrying off to the next thing that needs to be done.

Integrated with the Intellectual Eater

When these two worlds blend it means that the Functional Eater needs to start *thinking* about what they're eating, rather than just tasting it. This can be quite a leap for the Functional Eater to make in their mindset around food, but it's important as it can often mean the difference between the Functional Eater eating healthily and unhealthily. As such, the Functional Eater would usually rather attend a lecture or watch a DVD to learn about health than read a book – it takes less time! Even better would be some menu plans that tell them exactly what to eat to get everything they need, and someone to prepare those meals.

Integrated with the Emotional Eater

This combination is not the best because it leads to erratic unhealthy eating and, potentially, bingeing. This is because the Functional Eater does not usually take the time to make healthy, tasty food and so, when mixed with emotion, they would just grab things – anything – and this could lead to some pretty distasteful combinations and habits forming that would not be healthy for body, mind or soul. See the Emotional Eater section (pages 47–57) for more about how to break free from destructive eating habits.

Integrated with the Focused Eater

These two can work powerfully well together as long as the Functional Eater is supported with the specific foods and drinks they need to reach their goals easily and with minimum fuss. For the sports-orientated, this would show up as pre-packaged shakes, ready meals and protein bars. For those wishing to lose weight it would be the pre-prepared slimming meals and the menu plans all mapped out with rules and guidelines. Because the Functional Eater is non-emotional about food, generally speaking, they are the perfect candidates for integrating with the Focused Eater successfully.

Integrated with the Intuitive Eater

When these two types blend it's an interesting one, as the Functional Eater has to stop and feel... both of which can be a challenge! Once they have got used to that, it's then a case of having to have a wide range of foods available and having recipes or combinations that are quick and easy to make and still 'hit the spot'. This is entirely achievable, but will mean that the Functional Eater will probably need to get adept at working with raw foods rather than cooked in order to get healthy, make foods quickly (a blender will become their new best friend), and also stay connected intuitively to have the best of both worlds.

Integrated with the Conscious Eater

This is a good mix because it won't mean a radical change, just making different and informed food choices. Because the Functional Eater is usually not attached to any particular foods in an addictive kind of way, once they know what's on and off the menu (as a result of their new consciousness around food), they just tweak existing habits accordingly and off they go again – except this time they feel emotionally happier about what they are eating. (They'll still be looking for it all to be mapped out for them, though!)

Integrated with the Experimental Eater

These two types both love being waited on, so this is an entirely easy fit, especially because the Experimental Eater tends to obtain a lot of their foods from places where it's pre-prepared or served up directly. When these two mix you can expect to see trips to unusual restaurants or multi-cultural shopping venues. When it comes to fast eating at home, the fridge will be lined with the more exotic items, but they'll still be good to go in less than 15 minutes.

Integrated with the Confused Eater

As with the Emotional Eater, this is not the best combination for peace in body, mind or soul. When the Functional Eater integrates with the Confused Eater, it can easily lead to highly disordered eating and poor food choices. This can then lead to frustration and eating issues. For this reason the Functional Eater will work best with those types that add depth, clarity or passion, for a better rounded experience and to bring a healthy dose of joy and appreciation to the table. Generally speaking, no long-standing Functional Eater welcomes the possibility of integrating with the Confused Eater – they simply don't have the time or inclination to make food any more time-consuming or energy-consuming than it already is.

Integrated with the Social Eater

It goes without saying that this is a match made in heaven, providing the social situations serve the kinds of meals that the Functional Eater wants to eat. With food on tap via dinner parties, restaurants, barbecues and all manner of social situations, the Functional Eater is free to enjoy the 'done for you' element of eating while having great experiences to boot. In some cases, however, this heaven can turn to hell if the social situations they get involved with are not in alignment with any personal preferences the Functional Eater may have, such as quality, purity or ethical concerns around the food, in which case the social situations they engage with will need to be handpicked or pre-prepared for in order to avoid internal or external conflict.

The Conscious Evolution of the Functional Eater

The Functional Eater is primarily tuned in to their body (specifically their hunger) – that's it!

- **In its weakest expression:** can lead to poor health, lack of energy and even nutritional deficiencies (through junk food choices made for speed and taste).

- **In its highest expression:** you could have a very healthy, pre-prepared diet that is nutritionally sound as well as physically satiating.

The ultimate evolution for the Functional Eater is to move beyond eating purely to live and feel full, and join in the fun and depth that food has to offer by embodying the following Eater Types: Sensual + Intellectual + Conscious + Intuitive + Focused.

When the Functional Eater does this, they create the experience of:

- having food that is quick to eat and go

- loving the food they eat

- knowing that what they are eating is good for them

- feeling genuinely happy with their food choices from an ethical standpoint

- being more tuned in to their body and what *it* wants

- reaching and maintaining their personal body goals.

See pages 253–55 for some great food ideas for the healthy Functional Eater.

SIGNATURE DISH FOR THE FUNCTIONAL EATER
the green smoothie

The Green Smoothie is the perfect choice for the Functional Eater because it takes three minutes to make, uses just two ingredients, can easily be considered a meal in and of itself, and will give them energy and taste to fuel them up for the next exciting activity.

Serves   1–2

Equipment   Blender

Ingredients 1 large sweet and ripe mango (or 2 small ones)
5–6 large handfuls of spinach

Directions

• Chop your peeled mango into pieces and put into a blender (it's important that you put the mango in first, as it creates the juice which the spinach can be blended into).

• Wash your spinach thoroughly and add to the blender.

• Blend the two together until a thick, smooth consistency is achieved.

• Taste-test: if it's not sweet enough for you, add 1–2 dates or more mango. If it's too sweet, add a bit more spinach.

• Finally, if you prefer your smoothie less thick, simply add water to reach desired consistency.

• When you're happy with taste and texture, pour into a tall glass and swoon. Feel the green goodness flooding into you!

KAREN'S TIP

I recommend that you make 2 pints' worth (the above recipe will make roughly this amount) and drink one immediately and put the other into a pint glass and keep in the fridge until later in the day. The latter makes for a great afternoon 'snack' or satiating pre-dinner filler. Two in a day? It's super-efficient, doesn't take any extra time to make and you'll be feeling so much better in no time at all!

THE SENSUAL EATER 🍎

Sensual Eaters are generally passionate about many things, and food is one of them. They love to engage with what they eat and drink in a deeper and richer way than most people, and when they are eating they feel as if they are doing more than simply that – it's more of an experience, something that enhances their life. (The Sensual Eater will be the one who looks like they're in a world of their own when they're eating – they generally are!) Even if they feel conflicted about what they are eating, knowing that it may not be good for their health or waistline, they will still love being seduced by it. For the Sensual Eater, it is all about pleasure and feeling indulged.

The Sensual Eater's view –

- on food: 'Gorgeous'

- on eating: 'Pleasurable'

- on self-catering: 'Fun'

- on takeaways: 'Yum'

- on being personally catered for: 'Heaven'

- on eating out: 'Yippee!'

- on changing their diet: 'As long as it's delicious and I don't feel deprived, then I'm open to the possibility… maybe.'

The Sensual Eater and Pleasure

Sensual Eaters love it when…

- **their food feels decadent or 'naughty'.** You will generally find the Sensual Eaters at the chocolate tastings, cake shop or deli counter, clearly identifiable from the mischievous and excited glint in their eye. Healthier Sensual Eaters will seek out the most decadent varieties of whatever goes, according to their dietary bent – raw chocolate, vegan

24

cookies and higher-ticket organic staples – which serve even more to feed their desire for indulgence.

- **they discover something new and delicious.** Forever the pleasure-seeker, the Sensual Eater adores it when a new food comes into their world that they can go gaga over. It gives them something else to dream and fantasize about, and gives their world a whole new dimension.

- **they find the ultimate win–win for them – scrumptious AND sexy!** Sensual Eaters often make for sensual lovers because of their almost constant desire to 'feel' and experience pleasure. Having a body that they love and feel proud of affords them even *more* pleasure as they get to indulge in another way of being physical that is usually just as important to them as food. So finding a way of eating that enables them to look and feel their best, while not compromising on taste or decadence, is their ultimate dream.

The Sensual Eater's idea of heaven: 'Strawberries dipped in chocolate in one hand, a glass of champagne in the other, and an attractive lover at my side eager to get sensual with me.'

The Sensual Eater and Pain

Sensual Eaters struggle when…

- **food starts to get serious.** The Sensual Eater's worst nightmare is being told or finding out that they can't consume a favourite food or drink anymore. Not only does it induce feelings of deprivation but it also challenges them at the fundamental level of their identity. Who would they be if they didn't have their life and thoughts revolve around food anymore? This is entirely workable, but the Sensual Eater also has to be prepared to grow as a person to find new ways that work.

- they don't have access to anything other than basic, low-budget food. Not all Sensual Eaters are obsessed about quality, but what they do all have in common is that they can't bear food to be plain – this is only OK in emergency situations! So being in a situation where food is dull, low-key or basic in any way simply doesn't work for them. It's like someone has taken away their air supply.

- their partner doesn't share the same excitement about food. If two Sensual Eaters get together then naturally they'll adore and appreciate each other's foodie inclinations, and it could very well be the glue that binds them. This is all well and good and could be a match made in heaven – however, just as likely, if not more so, is that they both become seriously overweight and/or their life starts revolving around food 24/7 – that's if they get out of bed, of course! When the Sensual Eater chooses a mate who isn't quite as excited about what's for dinner, this has its share of struggles, but these can be overcome if both parties bring in a little bit of each other's dominant type so that they can find a place of balance and harmony which benefits them equally.

The Sensual Eater's idea of hell: 'Being fed a diet of cheap white bread and spam sandwiches for breakfast, lunch and dinner for a week.'

If This Is You

If you are a Sensual Eater or if this type is part of your profile, bookmark this page for a second and turn to Chapter 2 (page 126) where there are three short but revealing questions I'd like you to have a think about. These will help you get more in touch with how being a Sensual Eater works for you *and* can cause issues for you. You don't have to do anything with this information just yet, but don't skip it as it is vital. Take this opportunity to reflect on things; you may well have one or two 'Aha!' moments that could be of tremendous value to you. Once you've done that, come back to this page and keep reading.

* *

Case Study: Celia, 45, Marbella

When Celia and I first met, she was feeling very disillusioned because, like many women, she felt she had tried every diet under the sun and each one had 'failed' her. Consequently, all of her most recent efforts to eat more healthfully and lose her excess weight were now very much half-hearted, and she had all but given up hope of ever regaining her once youthful, sexy body.

I explained to Celia that there was nothing wrong with her. I explained how, as a Sensual Eater (which was obvious from just speaking with her, but the quiz soon validated this for us), she was always going to want things that were 'naughty' or indulgent – it was part of her very being, and how most diets were simply not designed for the Sensual Eater, so she would most likely never find what she was looking for 'out there'.

This was music to Celia's ears because she had spent most of her adult life thinking that there was something wrong with her, and that she needed to be 'fixed'. She had never realized that she could find a way to celebrate and revel in her sensuality with food, and so had never even considered trying to work with it.

Together we spent some time running through all the foods and drinks that she loved to consume on a day-to-day basis, along with those she naturally migrated towards when eating socially or 'treating' herself. The good news was that she already loved some really healthy, low-fat foods and drinks, and genuinely wanted to consume them on a daily basis – it was the rest of the time that we needed to focus on, so that she could achieve a knock-out body and feel as if she were still honouring and enjoying her sensual side.

With some dedicated effort on both our parts, and some ongoing menu tweaking, within a month we had found the perfect plan for her to move forward with. To make the whole process easier and more fun, we worked with the energy of the Focused Eater to help her create a very specific and measurable vision of her ideal body that she could get truly excited about. Working with the energy of the Focused Eater also helped Celia to secure the inner accountability, standards and boundaries that were required to get her to her goal. Finally, just to ensure that the whole journey would be as pleasurable for Celia as the destination itself, we drew up a list of eight different highly indulgent yet non-edible treats that she had been denying herself. She then gave herself permission to give herself one of these (and they were very impressive!) every time she shed another 4 lb.

With all of these pieces in place, within three months Celia had lost an impressive 22 lb and reported feeling more gorgeous than she had for over 20 years! Although by the time our work together was complete she still had more weight to lose, she now had the plan and the means to get herself there, and she felt totally confident and positive that she could keep working it by herself. Celia had finally found her way.

. . . .

The Benefits of Being a Sensual Eater

- Brings more joy and appreciation in to your relationship with food.

- Allows you to take more time over your meals and savour them.

- Expands your appreciation of food and the finer things in life.

- Helps you to really taste food and dive deeper into your experience of taste.

- Enables you to explore the more indulgent side of yourself and see what's there.

Adopting the Habits of a Sensual Eater

- Take more time to prepare and eat food than usual – double it!

- Give time and attention to making your plate look attractive and enticing.

- Increase the amount of fancy or 'seductive' foods you buy and eat – and enjoy feeling 'naughty' when doing so.

- Treat yourself to an upscale dining experience and savour every mouthful.

- Reprogramme yourself to see food as something that nourishes you on many levels.

Integrating with Other Types

Integrated with the Functional Eater

When the Sensual Eater integrates with the Functional Eater, it's a very different experience indeed. Being used to eating for pleasure rather than hunger, the Sensual Eater can struggle to understand – let alone change – to eating out of need rather than desire, and quite frankly feels the Functional Eater must be mad. Having said that, when the Sensual Eater does start eating only when hungry, immediate and appreciated weight loss is usually the result and, overall, a greater sense of balance and putting food well and truly in its place.

Integrated with the Intellectual Eater

When these two worlds blend it means that the Sensual Eater needs to start *thinking* about what they're eating, rather than just enjoying it. This can be quite an ask for the Sensual Eater because a lot of the time they'd really rather not think about anything beyond how something makes them feel. It's important, however, as it usually makes the difference as to whether the Sensual Eater eats healthily or not. When the Sensual Eater decides to start questioning their food, they prefer to do it via a book while snuggled up on the sofa, eating something decadent but healthy. Ideally, though, they'd love to be with a partner who is either an Intellectual Eater or a Focused Eater, who can help them indulge but in a healthful way, knowing that they have done all the reading, investigating and thinking for them.

Integrated with the Emotional Eater

This combination is far from ideal, in fact it's the worst of all for the Sensual Eater because it creates an environment where gluttony, overeating and poor food choices will flourish and potentially create physical, emotional and spiritual mayhem. As they are already first-rate foodies anyway, Sensual Eaters certainly do not need any more prompting to indulge or eat unnecessarily, which is exactly what the Emotional Eater energy will do for them. In fact, Sensual Eaters can only thrive when they integrate with a type that is more evolved. For them, the Emotional Eater is not it.

Integrated with the Focused Eater

The Focused Eater is the best type of all for the Sensual Eater to integrate with because it prevents all the negatives of the Sensual Eater from taking effect. When these two co-exist it's the best of both worlds: extreme pleasure and impressive health results. A Sensual Eater who integrates with the Focused Eater can expect to discover a whole new world of food and eating that piques their interest in all things foodie *and* allows them to experience a relationship with their body, food and what's possible, all at the same time. Could it get any better than this? If your current dominant type is the Sensual Eater, then try it and see for yourself!

Integrated with the Intuitive Eater

This is a great fit for the Sensual Eater because the Intuitive Eater is another 'feeling'-based type which thrives on 'tuning in' to food, self and environment. By integrating with the Intuitive Eater, the Sensual Eater gets to evolve in a way that is fascinating to them. No longer do they operate within the (usually) one-dimensional bubble that they have got so used to; now they get to expand their senses into feeling beyond their immediate pleasure zone and into their greater self and the world at large. For the Sensual Eater who loves to open up to a deeper part of themselves, the Intuitive Eater is the most perfect fit for enabling them to evolve beyond their immediate five senses and into their sixth.

Integrated with the Conscious Eater

Most Sensual Eaters experience inner struggle and shortness of breath when considering integrating with the Conscious Eater! This is because the Sensual Eater usually avoids thinking too deeply (if at all) about where their food comes from, and the price that anyone or anything has had to pay in order that they can indulge their desires. So when 'reality' comes into the equation, a challenging conversation can ensue. This will only be a successful and rewarding integration if the Sensual Eater is ready to look honestly at what's on their plate and is prepared to make some changes. For those who do, a really special experience awaits. They will feel suitably awake, proud and responsible for what gets to go in their shopping bag and also for every other choice they make in their life. In short, they'll become an even more loving and lovable person as they extend their heart and compassion beyond their own private universe.

Integrated with the Experimental Eater

It is not a big ask for the Sensual Eater to integrate with the Experimental Eater, and often the two automatically co-exist anyway. For Sensual Eaters who tend to keep to the same 'tried and adored' foods because they know what they like, proactively integrating with the Experimental Eater can lead to whole new worlds of experience, enjoyment and who knows what? (Most Sensual Eaters would be very open to the 'who knows what?' possibility.) The downside to this new experience is that, unless there is a more evolved type in the mix (e.g. Intellectual, Focused, Conscious or Intuitive), this combination will not eradicate the downsides of being a Sensual Eater and may, in fact, exacerbate them.

Integrated with the Confused Eater

There is nothing to be gained by the Sensual Eater becoming confused! Sensual Eaters positively hate being confused at the best of times, and they will absolutely detest being confused in their eating habits. Needless to say, this is *not* a recommended integration. The only time the Sensual Eater is likely to somewhat willingly integrate with the Confused Eater is when they are transitioning to an identity that is more evolved and therefore potentially challenging. At that point, as they mentally, emotionally or spiritually wrangle with new information and possibilities, they may automatically find themselves spending time and energy hanging out with the Confused Eater as they try to piece together their new way of being around food in a more evolved chapter of their life.

Integrated with the Social Eater

The Sensual Eater generally always loves to eat out – unless it's somewhere that's ugly, dirty, poorly presented, has a bad reputation or, of course (heaven forbid) where the menu is dull.

For the Sensual Eater who integrates with the Social Eater, life can quickly become one big party – and for many Sensual Eaters, the first thing that would spring to mind in this new reality would be 'This is the life!' This is great and definitely the case if the Sensual Eater's main desire is to have more fun, indulgence and camaraderie around food. However, if they're looking for something different with more depth and meaning, then they need to turn their attention to integrating with the types listed below, keeping the Social Eater as a type that they have some fun with now and again when they need to throw off any perceived shackles and indulge their naughty side.

The Conscious Evolution of the Sensual Eater

The Sensual Eater is tuned in to body, heart and soul.

- **In its weakest expression:** can lead to disrespect for the body and being overweight when the focus is not on what is good for the cells, but only on what tastes and/or feels good.

- **In its highest expression:** you could have a fabulously romantic, deeply pleasurable and impressively respectful relationship with food, where moderation prevents most of the downsides that could occur if you were to overindulge or remain insular about your food.

The ultimate evolution for the Sensual Eater is to wake up and embody the following Eater Types: Intellectual + Conscious + Intuitive + Focused.

When the Sensual Eater does this they create the experience of:

- loving the food they eat
- knowing that what they are eating is good for them
- feeling genuinely happy with their food choices from an ethical standpoint

- being more tuned in to their body and what *it* wants

- reaching/maintaining their personal body goals.

See pages 253–55 for some great food ideas for the healthy Sensual Eater.

SIGNATURE DISH FOR THE SENSUAL EATER

fresh strawberries dipped in raw chocolate sauce

This treat is the perfect choice for the Sensual Eater because it is beautiful to look at, tastes divine, feels naughty and is the perfect dish to share with a lover.

Serves 1–2

Equipment Food processor

Ingredients Fresh strawberries (as many as you desire)

1 cup raw cacao powder (cocoa powder also works but may be stronger)

1 cup agave nectar

Directions

- Wash your fresh strawberries well, taking care to leave the stalks on. (Sensual Eaters like the contrast!)

- Put your cacao powder and agave syrup into the food processor and blend until you have a thick, smooth, chocolaty mixture that is the same consistency all the way through.

- Place your strawberries in a medium-sized bowl and pour the chocolate dipping sauce into a smaller bowl in the middle.

- Enjoy by simply dipping the strawberries into the sauce and eating/ sharing/feeding as many or few as desired.

KAREN'S TIP

This sauce keeps brilliantly in the fridge for a few weeks, so make as much as you want and enjoy!

THE INTELLECTUAL EATER 🍎

For the Intellectual Eater, tasty food is great, but having it make sense and be the 'correct' way to eat is much more important – they need to feel that they are eating in the best way possible nutritionally and to understand fully how and why this is so. You will often find the Intellectual Eater reading a nutritional textbook or scientific-based food book. Eating for pleasure is seen as insane behaviour!

Intellectual Eaters are passionate about doing the right thing and feeding their body in the best possible way, sometimes even if they don't necessarily like what they are consuming. For the Intellectual Eater it is all about doing the research and doing the 'right thing'.

The Intellectual Eater's view –

- on food: 'Nutrition'
- on eating: 'Necessary'
- on self-catering: 'Fine'
- on takeaways: 'Pass'
- on being personally catered for: 'Ideal'
- on eating out: 'Challenging'
- on changing their diet: 'If it's an improvement on what I'm doing now, then I'm all for it, but I have to be convinced.'

The Intellectual Eater and Pleasure

Intellectual Eaters love it when…

- **they find a healthier alternative to something they have always loved eating.** Intellectual Eaters love discovering a new superfood or supplement that will take their diet to the next level or simply tick the right boxes. While they are not usually foodies in any way, shape or form, they do love to be able to find super-nutritious alternatives to things that they enjoy but know could be improved upon.

- **they discover some new cutting-edge information.** The Intellectual Eater loves that nutritional science is continually evolving, as there is always something new and exciting to learn – about both food and their body. This is why the best thing you could possibly give an Intellectual Eater for their birthday would be a metabolic type testing or food sensitivity test so that they can fine-tune their diet even more.

- **they feel they have it all figured out.** The moment the Intellectual Eater feels that they have everything figured out and they know exactly what to eat, when and why, is literally one of the best moments of their life.

The Intellectual Eater's idea of heaven: 'All my menus mapped out for me to give me everything I need nutritionally, and a personal chef who will make it all for me every day.'

The Intellectual Eater and Pain

Intellectual Eaters struggle when...

- **things get confusing.** The Intellectual Eater strives for absolute confidence and clarity in whatever it is that they read or discover, because once these are in place they can take action. With action comes peace and, hopefully, results. So when they come across conflicting, woolly or unsubstantiated information, their whole being can literally feel shattered. It's as if the whole world has been turned upside down, and they will do anything to get it feeling like it all makes sense again.

- **something they thought would work simply isn't working.** Unfortunately for Intellectual Eaters, they do have to learn at some point that we are way more complex than just being a sum of our parts. While the numbers may add up on the calculator, the results may not be so cut and dried in real life. While this can be a confusing and frustrating realization, it does pave the way for whole-person evolution, which is ultimately a very good thing indeed.

- **they can't find their ideal food path.** The Intellectual Eater's overriding quest is to find the ultimate way of eating or, at the very least, the ultimate way of eating for them. Every research paper read, every food experimented with, every label studied, all of it is done with just one main goal in mind: to find and eat that single most perfect diet. When this doesn't come together it can turn the Intellectual Eater into a Confused Eater, and unless they evolve on other levels or hit upon something that makes complete and utter sense to them (and works), this unfortunately can end up being where they stay.

    The Intellectual Eater's idea of hell: 'Not knowing what's best for me to eat at this stage of my life and not knowing where to look.'

If This Is You

If you are an Intellectual Eater or the Intellectual Eater is part of your profile, bookmark this page for a second and turn to Chapter 2 (page 126), where I'd like you to have a think about three short (but revealing!) questions. These will help you get more in touch with how being an Intellectual Eater has worked for you *and* how it has caused issues for you. You don't have to do anything with this information just yet, but don't skip it as it is vital. Take this opportunity to reflect on things; you may well have one or two 'Aha!' moments that could be of tremendous value to you. Once you've done that, come back to this page and keep reading.

Case Study: Robert, 49, Chichester

When I first spoke to Robert it was clear to me right away that he was an Intellectual Eater because of his constant references to the nutritional profiles of various foods, and whether he considered something to be good for him or not.

It was no surprise, then, to learn that Robert's goal was to find the healthiest possible way of eating for himself. He felt confident that he had a fairly good handle on food and nutrition, but thought that there was always room for improvement and he wanted to find out exactly what that was. In particular he wanted to find out more about raw foods, about which he had only a limited amount of knowledge.

While I was more than happy to help Robert with his goal, something he said in our initial conversation suggested to me that there was actually more that he wanted from his diet but he just wasn't saying it. In fact, I had a feeling that even he didn't realize that he wanted it, and so I ventured, *'Robert, I really get that you want to find the healthiest possible way of eating for you and I can certainly help you explore the world of raw foods as part of that quest, but I'm wondering: how much enjoyment do you actually get from food? Do you actually like eating?'*

Robert went quiet for a moment, and then replied, *'That's a very good question. You know, I hadn't really thought about it before, but no, I probably don't enjoy eating all that much actually. I just see it as something that I have to do and so I want to make sure that what I'm eating is as good as it can be.'*

I totally understood Robert's stance, especially as four out of five of his answers had come out as those of an Intellectual Eater (the fifth was that of a Focused Eater – hence his determination). Both of these types are thought-led rather than feeling-led, so it was no surprise to me that he hadn't stopped to consider whether what he was eating actually brought him any degree of happiness or pleasure.

After a conversation about this, Robert decided that he *did* want to consciously factor in receiving more pleasure from his diet because he saw some wisdom and benefit in that, although it transpired that he was equally resistant, too, because he feared he might 'let it all hang out and go the other way.' After enquiring where this fear came from I soon discovered that he had grown up with a father who was very much a Sensual Eater whose indulgence knew no bounds, and who had sadly died young from a heart attack because of it. I assured him that becoming a fully fledged Sensual Eater was *extremely*, if not *completely*, unlikely in his case, considering how strong his mental focus was around his diet, so he would be wise to shelve his concerns, at least for the short term, and to take this side of his work with me in small, low-impact steps.

This approach sat well for him, and our work together proved very fruitful, especially because the new path I took him on with raw foods proved to be incredibly fascinating and exciting to him. With this new and increased knowledge and passion for nutrition, Robert found that he also didn't seem quite so scared to start enjoying his food. In fact, this started happening naturally. He discovered that the quality raw foods and superfoods he was eating tasted so much better to him than many of the other 'healthy' foods he had been almost force-feeding himself, that he felt he had finally found his best of all possible worlds.

. . . .

The Benefits of Being an Intellectual Eater

- Using your mind and/or science to help you define your food choices.

- Having deeper understanding about what it is that you're eating.

- Learning more about the nutritional properties of foods.

- Learning more about how your body works, specifically in conjunction with diet.

- Moving away from your heart and into your head around food.

Adopting the Habits of an Intellectual Eater

- Choose a food-related topic you want to learn more about and start researching it like a scientist.

- Work out a week's menu from a calorie/nutrient perspective and try to reach every RDA.

- Study human physiology, and specifically anything and everything to do with digestion, absorption and elimination.

- Seek to create the healthiest possible eating plan for yourself.

- Aim to create the most nutrition-packed recipes each time you make a drink or meal.

Integrating with Other Types

Integrated with the Functional Eater

The Intellectual Eater is a naturally good match for the Functional Eater, as both are non-emotional about food and can be very matter-of-fact about it. If the Intellectual Eater is looking to create a food routine or lifestyle that is efficient and low-maintenance, then integrating with the Functional Eater will get them there. The downside of this integration is that the Functional Eater is not usually at all bothered about the nutrient content of their meals, so unless you are looking simply to speed up and get a more streamlined routine, then integrating with the Functional Eater would not be the best integration for you.

Integrated with the Sensual Eater

This particular integration can be a very interesting and expansive one for the Intellectual Eater as they get to start *experiencing* food rather than just thinking about it and eating it. As the Sensual Eater is all about using the senses to explore and enjoy food – terrain that the Intellectual Eater is typically not interested in – this can round out both the mindset and the overall experience of the Intellectual Eater in ways that will at first make them uneasy, and then will either open them up to a more diverse and sensory-driven diet, or make them stick to their guns even more and remain firmly of the opinion that using your brain around what you eat is a much more sane path than eating whatever tastes good.

Integrated with the Emotional Eater

There is nothing to be gained by the Intellectual Eater integrating with the Emotional Eater, as it would only ever be a backwards step. However, this could come about if the Intellectual Eater goes through a turbulent time in their life and suddenly stops caring about what is going into their body – in emotionally driven-sized portions. The good news is that, even if this should happen, the Intellectual Eater is so good at rationalizing things generally that they will quickly find a way to extricate themselves from this 'living hell' and simply address whatever has upset them in a proactive, 'get it sorted' kind of way.

Integrated with the Focused Eater

This pairing is one of the best of all, as both the Intellectual Eater and the Focused Eater are very results-orientated and like to use food to serve a specific outcome. What's especially helpful about the Intellectual Eater integrating with the

Focused Eater is that the Focused Eater is first-rate at being really clear about what's allowed and what's not. Sometimes the Intellectual Eater doesn't always have that level of clarity or parameters that are narrow enough to pinpoint when anything specific happens, so this integration will lead to an evolution that ensures that all of the Intellectual Eater's study and diligence will translate into something measurable and meaningful, which is what they've secretly been hankering for, anyway.

Integrated with the Intuitive Eater

This is not necessarily an easy integration for the Intellectual Eater to make, as the Intuitive Eater likes to feel their way through things, rather than think. However, when the Intellectual eater gets clear on what foods are considered OK and then eats intuitively within those parameters, it can be wonderfully liberating to start eating instinctively rather than constantly assessing if they've eaten enough protein/carbs/fat/calories/whatever each day. For Intellectual Eaters who are ready to evolve and start trusting their body more to see what happens, this is the specific integration that will get them there.

Integrated with the Conscious Eater

This combination is not too much of a stretch for the Intellectual Eater if they feel confident that they will still get everything that they need nutritionally. For this to work, the Intellectual Eater will need to do thorough research to prove to themselves that the path they are choosing will not harm them or leave them nutritionally deficient in any way. Once this has been established then you would be hard pressed to find a more passionate, committed and persuasive Conscious Eater.

Integrated with the Experimental Eater

The combination would work really well and for the better as the Experimental Eater has the potential to bring in even more new and beneficial foods, recipes and ingredients to the Intellectual Eater's diet, which they can then get really excited about. This is an easy integration to make as the Intellectual Eater is wired to seek, and is always looking for 'more', so the pioneering spirit of the Experimental Eater is sure to keep bringing in a steady supply of new and powerful superfoods and nutrient-dense goodies.

Integrated with the Confused Eater

As with the Emotional Eater, this is not an integration that the Intellectual Eater would be wise to choose willingly, as it won't get them where they want to be and will instead cause only stress, anxiety and suffering. It is not uncommon for the Intellectual Eater to integrate with the Confused Eater at various intervals on their path, however, as in their quest to seek out the right and best information there will be times when they come across conflicting data, and confusion will be the result. Depending on the mental and emotional stability of the Intellectual Eater, this unwanted 'dalliance' with Confused Eating may last for anything from a few seconds to many years. The best course of action the Intellectual Eater can take to prevent this from happening is to hold tight to the things that they're totally convinced about and be OK with a lack of clarity in other areas, trusting that the true and correct answers will reveal themselves very soon.

Integrated with the Social Eater

As the Social Eater is typically only pleasure-driven, this is not a brilliant match. The Intellectual Eater often purposefully *avoids* eating out socially because, for the most part, they know that a restaurant, dinner party, café or any other eating venue is never going to deliver anything like what they want – at least not without an element of stress. The only times this would be a good integration would be when the Intellectual Eater wants to network with others of a like mind and eating healthfully is part of the deal, or when they are feeling socially bankrupt and believe that eating out is the only way they can access quality time with their friends, family, colleagues or partner.

The Conscious Evolution of the Intellectual Eater

The Intellectual Eater is tuned in to their body and mind.

- **In its weakest expression:** can lead to an over-obsession with food quality and nutrition, where the eating experience becomes completely soul-less, pleasure-less and one-dimensional.

- **In its highest expression:** you could be one of the healthiest, most glowing and vibrant people you know and be reaping the benefits of eating a high-nutrient, well-balanced diet.

The ultimate evolution for the Intellectual Eater is to wake up and embody the following Eater Types: Sensual + Conscious + Intuitive + Focused. When the Intellectual Eater does this they create the experience of:

- knowing that what they are eating is good for them

- loving the food they eat

- feeling genuinely happy with their food choices from an ethical standpoint

- being more tuned in to their body and what *it* wants

- reaching/maintaining their personal body goal.

See the list on pages 253–55 for some great food ideas for the healthy Intellectual Eater.

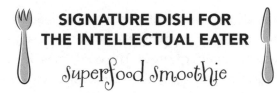

SIGNATURE DISH FOR
THE INTELLECTUAL EATER
Superfood Smoothie

This drink is really a meal and drink all in one. It's perfect for the Intellectual Eater as it's easy to digest, is great food-combining and is packed full of nutrients.

Serves   1

Equipment   Blender

Ingredients 1–2 large ripe bananas (use frozen bananas for a cooler, creamier drink)

1 tbsp Nature's Living Superfood or your favourite green superfood

2 cups pure water (or to desired consistency)

Dates to taste (optional; pre-soaked if dried; medjool or honey dates are the best and require no soaking)

Directions

• Simply blend all of the ingredients together until smooth. It takes just a few seconds and you're good to go!

KAREN'S TIPS

Feel free to ramp up the nutrition by adding any of your favourite superfoods of the moment. Good examples are hemp milk, seed or oil; chlorella; spirulina; chia seeds; ground flax; maca powder; sesame seeds.

If you make twice as much you can have one for breakfast and then either carry the rest to work in a flask or cooler or refrigerate the second half for when you get home.

THE EMOTIONAL EATER

The Emotional Eater is usually not a happy person around food because they're frequently in a state of angst about what they're eating. They tend to oscillate between 'treating' themselves and punishing themselves depending on what is going on in their life, and food is usually the main way in which to do this.

The Emotional Eater desperately wants to find a way of eating that brings them harmony and, because they search outside of themselves for the solution (rather than internally, which is where the situation needs to be addressed), they can find themselves yo-yo dieting in their bid to find the 'perfect' way. For the Emotional Eater, their story is usually about 'doing a dance' around food when really they should be spending their precious time and energy listening to their heart.

The Emotional Eater's view –

- on food: 'Comforting'

- on eating: 'Painful'

- on self-catering: 'Dangerous'

- on takeaways: 'Risky'

- on being personally catered for: 'Helpful'

- on eating out: 'Enjoyable'

- on changing their diet: 'If it stops me overeating and helps me to control my eating, then I'll give it a whirl.'

The Emotional Eater and Pleasure

Emotional Eaters love it when…

- they think that they have found a way of eating that will finally bring them the peace they are seeking. Emotional

Eaters want nothing more than to find the magic way that will bring them peace and harmony around food. Because they typically believe that the solution begins and ends with food and a certain way of eating, their search can go on for years or even decades until they do indeed find a way of eating that enables them to come into balance and develop healthy eating patterns – but it certainly won't be a one-dimensional solution when it comes.

- **they have a day when they don't eat for emotional reasons and feel in control of their eating.** This kind of day for the Emotional Eater is a very happy day indeed. Sometimes they are rare, sometimes they come in clusters, but when they come it's a time where there is hope and the possibility of another way of being around food – and the perfect opportunity to see what's different that has made this experience possible.

- **they have any kind of breakthrough around why they're overeating, and feel that an end to their struggle might be in sight.** Some Emotional Eaters are aware that they are only going to be able to find their eating nirvana when they heal their heart or take care of whatever is bothering them, but others are not quite so aware. Either way, when they have any kind of 'Aha!' moment around their behaviour and start to feel a new level of understanding or possibility for themselves, this moves them closer to their desired destination and is a wonderful moment indeed.

The Emotional Eater's idea of heaven: 'When I don't overeat or don't eat badly for more than a week.'

The Emotional Eater and Pain

Emotional Eaters struggle when…

- **they have 'a bad day'.** The Emotional Eater tends to talk in terms of 'good' and 'bad' a lot of the time because this is the yardstick that they tend to measure themselves by. Part of the issue lies in the language that they use, because it feeds their negative self-talk – which only serves to intensify the problem. Thus it becomes very easy for one 'bad day' to lead to another.

- **they thought they had 'cracked it' but it's all gone wrong again.** There are always going to be some days that are better than others for the Emotional Eater, and these are the days that get them excited, but the not-so-great days that usually tend to follow bring them back down into the 'this is never going to happen for me' funk – which leads to more of the above.

- **they start believing that this is how it will always be.** It is very common and understandable for the Emotional Eater to buy into the belief that emotional eating is going to be their story for the rest of their life, because every day they accrue more evidence to support it. With no other story to buy into, no other 'plan' that they can believe in or actively follow, this is indeed the path that they are paving for themselves, but it doesn't have to be this way…

> *The Emotional Eater's idea of hell: 'Thinking that emotional eating is something I am never going to get over.'*

If This Is You

If you are an Emotional Eater, or this type is part of your profile, bookmark this page for a second, and turn to Chapter 2 (page 126), where I'd like you to consider three short but revealing questions. These will help you get more in touch with how being an Emotional Eater has worked for you *and* has caused you issues. You don't have to do anything with this information just yet, but don't skip it. It is vital, so do it now. Take this opportunity to reflect on things; you may well have one or two 'Aha!' moments that could be of tremendous value to you. Once you've done that, come back to this page and keep reading.

. . . .

Case Study: Samantha, 21, Melbourne

Samantha's history of emotional eating went way back to childhood, largely in response to a mother who used food in a multitude of ways: to cosset, calm, cajole and celebrate her four children all the way from babyhood to the present day.

In short, Samantha had the 'perfect' role model for emotional eating, and it was no wonder that her life had shaped up the way it had.

Although Samantha's mother apparently had no issue with her approach, by the time Samantha reached puberty, Samantha herself really did. Weight gain, spotty skin, low self-esteem and an inability to cope with stress without food all took their physical and emotional toll on Samantha, who, by the time she approached me, feared this would become the story of her life if she didn't address it head-on.

Thankfully, Samantha's emotional eating had not developed into any kind of significant eating disorder, however there were definitely times when she would consider herself very much out of control. From the very start it seemed as if this journey towards healing was going to be a long and winding road, but by working with the Eater Types it proved to be a lot easier than it might otherwise have been.

I got to know Samantha very well during our time together. Although food was what brought Samantha to me, at first most of our time was spent discussing everything except food. Once we had got clear on where Samantha really needed help to feel good about herself and life, we could then underpin our efforts with a food approach that worked well for who she was underneath the emotion, and that supported where she wanted to go. It was by working with the Functional, Intuitive and Focused Eater in her that we got her there.

Although it did take a lot of coaching and time to move things forward to a place where we both felt genuine progress had been made, by the time we were complete the changes were phenomenal. Not only was Samantha's emotional eating at an all-time low (just once every couple of weeks on average), but when she did comfort-eat it was controlled, genuinely pleasurable (as opposed to damaging) and she came out the other side of it feeling truly great about the way she had handled it.

Not only that, but she lost 14 lb in weight, her skin cleared up and she now had a plan for her life that genuinely excited her. Victory indeed!

. . . .

The Benefits of Being an Emotional Eater

It is rarely a good idea to consciously choose to move into being an Emotional Eater, unless it is considered an 'upgrade' from where you're currently at, or you're going to decide consciously to 'go there', 'own' it and use it as an opportunity to learn more about yourself in a controlled way (but you mustn't stay here for long, otherwise your plan will have backfired). The habits below will be helpful in helping you move beyond your Emotional Eater identity and will be even more powerful when combined with a different Eater Type profile and a helpful 'recipe for success' chosen from the options in Chapter 5.

Adopting the Habits of an Emotional Eater

*   Pay very close attention to what foods you are choosing and what messages they might have for you (e.g. sweet foods may indicate a need for more love or sweetness in your life; the need to bite into crunchy foods usually signals unexpressed anger).

- Pay attention to the severity and patterns around your emotional eating – what might they be telling you?

- Seek advice or therapy to help you learn to manage your emotions in healthy, non-damaging ways – with the intention of ridding yourself of any emotional reliance on food (this *is* achievable in time).

- Know that food will never solve a problem or mend a broken heart, and commit to finding ways that will.

Integrating with Other Types

Integrated with the Functional Eater

Integrating with the Functional Eater can be tremendously helpful for the Emotional Eater due to the Functional Eater's unemotional, matter-of-fact approach to food. By eating according to the Functional Eater's number-one mantra – 'I only eat when I'm hungry' – the Emotional Eater is given the opportunity to become unavoidably aware of all the times that they are eating out of their emotional state. Providing they use this as a springboard for awareness and healing, and not as yet another opportunity to beat themselves up, this can be the single most powerful combination for illumination and lasting change. Only choose this combination when you feel truly ready to evolve out of your Emotional Eater identity and into something better, otherwise it will feel like a self-imposed bootcamp and could backfire spectacularly.

Integrated with the Sensual Eater

For the Emotional Eater, integrating with the Sensual Eater could be seen as a step up – but only just! Both types are emotionally driven, but the Sensual Eater is generally more stable in their eating habits, so when the Emotional Eater gives themselves permission to keep eating for pleasure but with certain boundaries in place, this could pave the way for a transition into more healthful eating patterns without undue stress. To guarantee true success, however, the Emotional Eater will need either to integrate another type *as well*, or move beyond the Sensual Eater stage completely in favour of one of the more unemotional types (Intellectual, Focused, Functional) to reach the desired destination of peace, poise and emotional mastery.

Integrated with the Intellectual Eater

This combination can be a great strategic move on the part of the Emotional Eater who wants to move out of their heart and into their head around food. By making food choices intellectually they automatically will make it difficult for themselves to justify eating certain things, especially those things which they know are not doing them any good. For the Emotional Eater who is overweight, integrating with the Intellectual Eater will typically lead to speedy and impressive weight loss. This can be just what the Emotional Eater needs to show them that they can indeed move forward and create a new reality for themselves without having to go through emotional drama to get there.

Integrated with the Focused Eater

As per combining with the Functional Eater, for the Emotional Eater to integrate with the Focused Eater some really big shifts need to occur. While many of these will be on the outside, with different food choices and habits being made, 75 per cent of it will need to be on the inside for the Emotional Eater to be able to stay strong, stable and focused in order to leave their old ways behind. Again, this is a step to be taken only when the Emotional Eater is truly ready for a breakthrough, except – surprisingly, perhaps – that integrating with a

Focused Eater will be more plain sailing than migrating across to being a Functional Eater, because the Emotional Eater's strong feelings can be channelled into helping them reach a specific, realistic and achievable goal. And then another, then another. This is the most sensible and effective path for the Emotional Eater who is ready to move on purposefully.

Integrated with the Intuitive Eater

This is an interesting integration for the Emotional Eater to make, as the Intuitive Eater is also a high-intensity feeling type. The way this can work, and it can work beautifully too, is if the Emotional Eater agrees 'I can eat anything that I want, but the directions must come from my body and I must stop when I'm full.' As you can appreciate, this gives the Emotional Eater the freedom that they are used to having but with helpful direction and boundaries. As a result of this integration, the Emotional Eater can evolve into eating only when hungry, eating what the body (not the heart) asks for and using the emotional poise they gain in the process to address the emotions that will inevitably come up.

Integrated with the Conscious Eater

Integrating with the Conscious Eater is helpful, to a point, as the Emotional Eater is usually extremely empathetic, which is why they can become an Emotional Eater in the first place. So, eliminating certain foods based on ethical, spiritual, moral and/or environmental considerations can move the Emotional Eater out of self-preoccupation and into thinking of the bigger picture and focusing on others. This attention-point shift can be a powerful tool for directing their powerful emotional energy out of their own bubble and into helping others, which is one of the most potent tools for healing, evolution and spiritual transformation known to humanity.

Integrated with the Experimental Eater

It is probably not the smartest move to integrate the Emotional Eater with the Experimental Eater, as there is not a lot to be gained by introducing yet more new foods and eating possibilities to the Emotional Eater who is trying to think less about food rather than more. Having said that, one way that this dynamic could work powerfully is to use the spirit of the Experimental Eater to try new ways of being around food, and literally experimenting with different ways of approaching food – from the inside. One example might be eating only between certain hours of the day. Another example might be eating only foods that are high water content (fresh fruits and vegetables) before noon. By being experimental about the process rather than about introducing new foods, this could be another transitional path that could help ease the Emotional Eater into something even more effective later.

Integrated with the Confused Eater

The last thing the Emotional Eater wants or needs is to be even more conflicted about food – they already have enough confusion going on around their emotions, without their mind being frustrated and mixed up too! For this reason, this integration is *not* recommended under any circumstances. What the Emotional Eater is ultimately crying out for is clarity. They need a framework that they can believe in and get excited about, and that works.

Integrated with the Social Eater

Emotional Eaters can swing between wanting to eat out often (for the emotional uplift that socializing can bring) and wanting to hide away and eat in secret without limitations. Integrating with the Social Eater could actually be a very smart move for the Emotional Eater if they decide that they will only eat when in the presence of others, because it will make their eating more ordered in terms of scheduling, and also more limited in quantity. This is one of those combinations where the structure that's put in place could lead to success, and also provide the companionship that could give the Emotional Eater the opportunity to share what's at the heart of their eating disharmony.

The Conscious Evolution of the Emotional Eater

The Emotional Eater is tuned in to their emotions and, to varying degrees, their soul.

- **In its weakest expression:** can spiral into increasing levels of food addiction, overweight and self-harm.

- **In its highest expression:** you may occasionally eat for comfort or to numb-out, like just about everyone else, but that is the rare exception rather than the rule.

The ultimate evolution for the Emotional Eater is to shift completely and embody the following Eater Types: Sensual + Intellectual + Conscious + Intuitive + Focused.

When the Emotional Eater does this they create the experience of:

- loving the food they eat (and finding their comfort within sensuality)

- knowing that what they are eating is good for them

- feeling genuinely happy with their food choices from an ethical standpoint

- being more tuned in to their body and what *it* wants

- reaching/maintaining their personal body goals.

See pages 253–55 for some great food ideas for the healthy Emotional Eater.

SIGNATURE DISH FOR
THE EMOTIONAL EATER

date surprises

This healthy recipe is a delicious and comforting treat/snack that has both sweetness and crunch for those times when you want to comfort-eat but don't want to feel bad about what you're eating.

Serves 1

Equipment None

Ingredients 4 medjool dates (or as many as you want to make!)

4–8 almonds or Brazil nuts

Directions

- Take your medjool dates, cut or rip them in half, de-stone them and place one or two almonds or Brazil nuts between the two halves.

KAREN'S TIP

Try any nut or filling in place of the almonds or Brazils. These two options are great but they're certainly not the only choices.

THE FOCUSED EATER 🍎

The Focused Eater is on a mission. Whether it's to lose weight, get fit, create the best life or find the perfect career or soulmate, they know where they're going and why, and my goodness they're going to get there! With the Focused Eater you can bet that everything they do, whether it's the food they eat or where they choose to place their other life energy, it is going to be 100 per cent aligned with whatever it is that they are going after – which is, of course, their recipe for success.

For the Focused Eater, life and food are exciting 'tools' that they work with because both get them exactly what they want. Yes indeed, for the most part at least, they've found the magic formula!

The Focused Eater's view –

- on food: 'Powerful'

- on eating: 'Pre-meditated'

- on self-catering: 'Perfect'

- on takeaways: 'Unlikely'

- on being personally catered for: 'Perfection'

- on eating out: 'Manageable'

- on changing their diet: 'Absolutely if it gets me even better results and gets me where I want to go faster.'

The Focused Eater and Pleasure

Focused Eaters love it when…

- **they come up with a new and exciting goal and a dietary plan to get them there.** Focused Eaters are naturally driven types, or evolve to become that way when a personal desire becomes all-consuming and of paramount importance. So naming and claiming a goal *and* finding the formula to get them there are among the things that make them thrilled to be alive.

- **they discover a new food or approach to eating that will enable them to get better, quicker or easier results than they are with their current *modus operandi*.** Focused Eaters love anything that helps them reach their goals more efficiently and/or joyfully. Even though they love the journey, their reasoning is that they're only really in it for the destination, and there are plenty of other destinations to be pursued after the next one has been reached, so why waste time cruising?

- **they reach one of their goals and they know exactly how and why it worked.** As analysis is one of the key secrets to Focused Eaters reaching their goals, to hit upon a winning combination that is guaranteed to work every time is like manna from heaven – which will not only be stored for future use if required, but will be used as a springboard to reach similar goals even faster than they otherwise would have been.

The Focused Eater's idea of heaven: 'Pursuing a goal with an eating plan that I know is going to get me there in a more powerful and effective way than ever before.'

The Focused Eater and Pain

Focused Eaters struggle when…

- **they don't have all the pieces.** The Focused Eater needs to know everything about everything, otherwise they can't get going because they feel ill-equipped for the journey. This is why you'll often find the Focused Eater closely intertwined with the Intellectual Eater (either within the same person or the company that they keep) because usually between them they manage to figure it all out.

- **things don't happen fast enough.** The Focused Eater's preferred speed in life is, quite simply, fast. This is because, once their mind is made up, they want what they want NOW. Sometimes being on Earth can feel way too slow for the Focused Eater, who is constantly wondering why the path of life was designed as long and winding rather than straight and narrow.

- **things don't go according to plan.** The Focused Eater is all about planning, so when something *doesn't* go to plan, it's frustrating to say the least! Still, Focused Eaters are never easily beaten, so you can bet that they will analyse what went wrong until they've got it all figured out. Once they have, they're up and off again and, one way or another, victory will be theirs!

The Focused Eater's idea of hell: 'Thinking that something around my eating is going to work fantastically to get me to my goal and then, for some reason, it simply doesn't.'

If This Is You

If you are a Focused Eater, or if this fits part of your Eater Type profile, bookmark this page for a second and turn to Chapter 2 (page 126), where there are three short (but revealing!) questions I'd like you to have a think about. These will help you get more in touch with how being a Focused Eater has worked for you *and* may have caused you issues. You don't have to do anything with this information just yet, but don't skip it; it is vital. Take this opportunity to reflect on things; you may well have one or two 'Aha!' moments that could be of tremendous value to you. Once you've done that, come back to this page and keep reading.

. . . .

Case Study: Simon, 38, Manchester

If anyone embodied the Focused Eater to its finest, it was Simon. He was the master of goal-setting (and goal-reaching!) and was one of the most positive, go-getting people you could ever hope to meet.

So it was with great surprise that I found Simon booking a call with me to discuss how I could help him. After all, this was a guy who coached others for a living and, as someone who had read and studied just about every personal and spiritual development guru on the planet, I thought he was the least likely type to need assistance with his food.

However, as with anyone, there is always room for improvement or another level of evolution to explore and, as I was soon to discover, Simon was no different.

Yes, he knew what to eat. Yes, he was master of his own domain and was as far away from an Emotional Eater as you could possibly get and, yes, he was usually pretty good at tuning in to his body and attending to its needs no matter what the situation. And, no surprise, he also had a body that he had every right to feel extremely proud of as a result. However, what Simon didn't have, and now really and truly wanted, was to feel authentically good on a deeper, more spiritual level about what and how he was eating. In short, he wanted to become more conscious.

Our work together was a lot of fun, and was soon completed, because Simon had a very open mind and was quick to implement whatever made sense to him. He was incredibly open to any suggestions I made about what 'conscious' might look like, although I stressed the importance of being aware that one person's idea of conscious can be very different from another's. So we spent some time exploring what conscious meant to *him*, and took that as our foundation on which to build.

During this time we covered a lot of ground – not only about food, but also about him as an individual and his life as a whole – because food and life are so inextricably linked. He soon became more conscious with his eating habits, and the deeper he went with that, the more this extended into *every* area of his life. He started making more conscious and fulfilling choices across the board.

By the time we had completed our work, not only had Simon established a way of eating that ticked all the boxes for him and that he could feel had spiritual integrity for him, he also had a new reverence for life and an even deeper worldview that brought him great joy on a personal level, and brought added benefits to *his* clients.

. . . .

The Benefits of Being a Focused Eater

- Reaching a very specific goal that needs you to modify your eating habits moderately or significantly.

- Becoming a lot more aware of what and how you eat.

- Learning more about your weaknesses around food.

- Putting more time and attention into what and how you are eating.

- Stepping into the ultimate level of mastery around your eating.

Adopting the Habits of a Focused Eater

- Set a very bold and specific goal for yourself that requires a high level of focus.

- From this moment, start becoming incredibly mindful about everything you think, do and feel around food.

- Work out an action plan for food and drink that will help you reach your goal.

- Create a list of alternative strategies to employ in the face of adversity or temptation.

- Get excited about holding yourself to the highest level of food mastery and what that could mean for you.

Integrating with Other Types

Integrated with the Functional Eater

The Focused Eater can benefit from integrating with the Functional Eater if they're looking to streamline their approach to food and eating. The Functional Eater will make things very matter-of-fact for the Focused Eater. There won't be any time for fluff or discussion. So the Focused Eater needs to draw up the rules and use their Functional Eater counterpart to put these rules into action as quickly as possible.

Where this integration would be a problem is if the Functional Eater part didn't follow the guidelines laid down by the Focused Eater. In this case the integration would lead to a downward spiral in standards, gratification and results.

Integrated with the Sensual Eater

The Focused Eater's world can be enhanced sensually if they integrate with the Sensual Eater, so long as, as for the Functional Eater integration, the Focused Eater is still calling the shots. By combining with the Sensual Eater, the Focused Eater stands to benefit from enjoying the journey as much as the destination, appreciating food more deeply on a sensual level, and discovering that taking the time to enjoy your food does not mean that your goal will take longer to achieve, but perhaps even the opposite.

Integrated with the Intellectual Eater

This combination is very common and effective because the two naturally collude on the same level, which is results-driven. Where the Intellectual Eater can be of service to the Focused Eater is via the former's desire to discover the facts, get them right and put them together in a formula that, at the very least, works on paper. The Focused Eater loves this as it's the firmest foundation on which to build, and will happily take that as the foundation for success and then continue to test and measure against what they are aiming for. And if the plan doesn't work, the Intellectual Eater will effectively be sent on a new fact-finding mission to get to the bottom of why the original plan was flawed.

Integrated with the Emotional Eater

The Focused Eater has nothing to gain by integrating with the Emotional Eater, other than to discover, just for a day, where their emotions may not be being supported if they suspect this is holding them back. This integration can also help them temporarily to let their undirected eating choices be the messenger or mirror for that. Once they get what they need, they should bid the Emotional Eater farewell, thank it for its input and act on the information collected so that their chances of success are now assured.

Integrated with the Intuitive Eater

The Focused Eater potentially has a lot to be gained from this integration, as the Intuitive Eater holds the capacity to 'tune in' to important information which may not be at all obvious, or even yet discovered. As the Intuitive Eater relies on their sixth sense to make eating decisions, it has the ability to flag up why something isn't working, or what's missing, which the Focused Eater has next to no chance of doing. For this reason, if the Focused Eater isn't getting the results expected despite rigorous testing and tweaking, it would be wise to integrate with the Intuitive Eater for a while to access information that could make all the difference.

Integrated with the Conscious Eater

The Focused Eater is usually not overly concerned with what the Conscious Eater has to say, as results are all that matter and they've bought into the belief that certain foods others might consider off-limits are necessary for their success. However, when the Focused Eater *does* choose to integrate with the Conscious Eater, what usually happens for them is the discovery that the same results (or even better ones) can be achieved through different and more conscious means. This can be such a revelation for the Focused Eater that they can become a huge proponent of conscious eating and very passionate about it. This is because, with their desire to be successful and to be the best in whatever they do at the heart of what drives them, if they can see a way to be ethically responsible in their winning formula, as well as reach their goals, then they're going to want to rave about it and spread the word.

Integrated with the Experimental Eater

The Focused Eater can benefit from integrating with the Experimental Eater in terms of discovering new foods, new approaches and new terrain to explore. This combination is a great way to go when the Focused Eater is ready to mix things up a bit, or even try something more extreme, unusual or outlandish. The spirit of the Experimental Eater will be sure to take them there!

Having said this, there does come a point in each individual pursuit where the mix may no longer be supportive, so the Focused Eater should be under no illusions that integrating with the Experimental Eater will result in helpful and less helpful times, and to stay mindful of when to let go of the relationship should it become unsupportive.

Integrated with the Confused Eater

The Focused Eater is bound to spend at least small amounts of time integrated with the Confused Eater because of their pioneering spirit. There will be times when plans do not work out, where things that seemed so certain come to nothing and where things that maybe worked before don't work the second time around. It's at this point that the Focused Eater runs the risk of falling into a relationship with the Confused Eater as it scratches its head in perplexity. So long as the confusion is used as a catalyst for coming to clarity as soon as possible, then all is not lost when this integration occurs.

Integrated with the Social Eater

The Focused Eater is famed for avoiding social situations which involve food because their needs are so specific that they hate the thought of coming off-track for anything or anyone. Indeed, one of the Focused Eater's hardest realities to bear is that most people love sharing food and mealtimes with others, and that it's a huge part of family life, human connection in general and society at large. For the Focused Eater who doesn't want to feel ostracized or alienated from their family or friends, they have the challenge of deciding exactly how they're going to integrate social eating with pursuing their goals.

The Conscious Evolution of the Focused Eater

The Focused Eater is tuned in to their body, heart, mind and soul – to varying degrees, depending on the individual.

- **In its weakest expression:** can become obsessive and neurotic, and unable to socialize happily or comfortably.

- **In its highest expression:** you are a fully-rounded and focused individual who has mastered food and eating in a way that most people are in complete awe of.

The ultimate evolution for the Focused Eater is simply to feel even better about the way they approach food while embodying the following Eater Types: Sensual + Intellectual + Conscious + Intuitive.

When the Focused Eater does this they create the experience of:

- loving the food they eat (which usually they could improve on, as they tend towards thinking rather than feeling)

- knowing that what they are eating is the best for them

- feeling genuinely happy with their food choices from an ethical standpoint

- being tuned in to their unique body and what *it* wants.

See pages 253–55 for some great food ideas for the healthy Focused Eater.

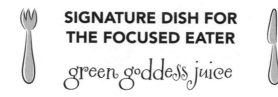

SIGNATURE DISH FOR THE FOCUSED EATER

green goddess juice

This drink is delicious, refreshing and super-healthy. When it comes to ticking all the boxes, this juice is perfect in every way and therefore perfectly perfect for the Focused Eater.

Serves 1–2

Equipment Juicer

Ingredients 200g organic spinach

5 sticks celery

1 whole cucumber, including peel

2 apples

1 medium (ripe) pineapple

½ a lemon, including its peel

½ a lime, including its peel

Directions

- Simply juice all of the ingredients in any order, pour into a jug and stir well.

KAREN'S TIPS

Keep in the fridge any you can't drink, and enjoy it cool later. This recipe keeps well owing to the lemon and lime, which help preserve it.

For an even more powerful drink, blend the juice with some high-quality bee pollen or spirulina powder.

THE INTUITIVE EATER 🍎

The Intuitive Eater is usually someone who has already walked a few different paths around food but has come to rest at a place of quiet and calm confidence which, generally speaking, is that 'the body knows best.' Intuitive Eaters are typically in a really good place with food and eating, with perhaps the odd detour depending on social, circumstantial or emotional reasons. For the Intuitive Eater, food is something to be enjoyed, but their first priority is always to listen to what their body is asking for; that consideration tends to trump every other one.

The Intuitive Eater's view –

* on food: 'Interesting'

* on eating: 'Pleasurable'

* on self-catering: 'Ideal'

* on takeaways: 'Unlikely'

* on being personally catered for: 'Problematic'

* on eating out: 'Fun'

* on changing their diet: 'I'm always changing my diet because I eat what my body tells me to.'

The Intuitive Eater and Pleasure

Intuitive Eaters love it when...

* **they feel the perfect union between what their body wants and what they give to it.** Intuitive Eaters live for the feeling of being connected, and the sweetest spot for them is when an extra-special level of connection is reached. This gets to happen for them when they are feeling clean, tuned in, spacious and relaxed, and they make their food choices from this picture-perfect place.

- **they make an impromptu 'guided' food choice and it ends up feeling magical.** Intuitive Eaters are much more likely to make an unexpected food choice from the produce aisle than any other type because they will literally tune in to food and be able to select – *even before eating* – exactly which food is right for them at that time. Intuitive Eaters are unique in that they have learned how to use all of their senses when selecting food, and their sixth sense is possibly the strongest of them all. When they make a choice from this place and the conditions are right, a feeling of magic and awe are inevitable.

- **they have a fridge full of food so they don't need to worry about not having enough to choose from.** Intuitive Eaters love and appreciate diversity because they never know exactly what they are going to want to eat ahead of time, and hate to be caught out. Having a range of foods that covers all different types of colours, flavours, textures and consistencies – and, typically, equal amounts of sweet and savoury foods – is an Intuitive Eater's dream and means they'll always find something they love to eat.

The Intuitive Eater's idea of heaven: 'When everything I eat feels perfect and every part of me feels centred, whole and aligned.'

The Intuitive Eater and Pain

Intuitive Eaters struggle when…

- **they see signs that they are starting to suffer from any kind of health-related issue.** Intuitive Eaters pride themselves on being so connected to their body that they feel they should never experience any kind of health concern. While the logic is understandable, the Intuitive Eater also knows that we, as humans, are multi-dimensional, and they are rational enough to know that while there may be a fault with their diet, it could just as easily be the result of imbalance in another aspect of their being.

- **they are feeling 'clogged up' internally and lack the connection with themselves that they seek.** Intuitive Eaters love to feel clean. It is this feeling of cleanliness that enables them to make the best food choices for themselves, as they are very in touch with what their body really wants. During times when their diet may not be so clean or ideal, their body can start to feel separate from them and connection is impaired. For this reason the Intuitive Eater will do well to incorporate a regular cleansing or fasting practice into their lifestyle to ensure that they can always feel confidently tuned in.

- **they are under stress and don't have time to shop, prepare or choose food in a way that feels good to them.** The Intuitive Eater isn't really one to faff about with food, as they generally like things clean and simple. However, when they don't have the time or space they need to get food in, tune in to themselves and gauge their feelings around food, their 'default setting' is to be Functional Eaters. This can have many negative knock-on effects.

The Intuitive Eater's idea of hell: 'Having to eat things that don't feel right and feeling out of kilter because of it.'

If This Is You

If you are an Intuitive Eater, or if this fits part of your Eater Type profile, bookmark this page for a second and turn to Chapter 2 (page 126), where there are three short (but revealing!) questions I'd like you to have a think about. These will help you get more in touch with how being an Intuitive Eater may work for you but also how it may cause issues for you at times. You don't have to do anything with this information just yet, but don't skip it; it is vital. Take this opportunity to reflect on things; you may well have one or two 'Aha!' moments that could be of tremendous value to you. Once you've done that, come back to this page and keep reading.

· ·

Case Study: Claire, 42, Utah

Claire came to me at a time when she was hugely frustrated with her eating habits, even though, historically, most of the time she'd been in a great, healthy and self-loving place with what and how she ate.

As a mostly Intuitive Eater, with a score of four out of five, and with Functional Eater scoring one, Claire had been used to being keenly in touch with her body and its needs, eating simply and cleanly most of the time. During recent times, however, this awareness seemed to be usurped by something else. Now, some months later, she found herself 10 lb overweight and feeling very out of touch with herself and her body, and the reality of the situation had finally called her into action.

Claire's goal was clear: she wanted to be back in touch with her true intuition and to lose the weight she had gained – but first we had to establish what had happened to get her off-kilter in the first place.

It transpired that Claire, a self-employed and highly successful businesswoman, had been under a lot of stress during the past year as her business had gone through a period of rapid expansion and her marriage had taken some strain during this time. Not only this, but as she put all her efforts into trying to manage the growth of her business *and* attend to her husband's needs, her own needs had been relegated to the bottom of the pile.

It soon became obvious why her food choices had become hurried, unsupportive and sometimes off-beam.

Now clearly seeing the connection, Claire immediately stopped giving herself a hard time and agreed with me that all of her attention, now that she was through the worst, should go back to herself and to reconnecting with her whole being so her Intuitive Eater could once again shine through.

Over the next few weeks we developed both a menu plan and a life plan that would help Claire create plenty of time for herself. Intuition needs space and peace to thrive, so she set about giving herself plenty of both – and it worked like a dream.

Now with sufficient space to hear her needs and honour them in a healthy way, the quick grab for the ice-cream tub immediately ceased, and within a very short space of time not only was Claire back in touch with her intuition, but the weight was easily falling away to reveal the authentic body, as well as soul, of a very wonderful woman.

. . . .

The Benefits of Being an Intuitive Eater

- Being able to tune in to your body and start listening with fresh and unbiased ears.

- Letting a deeper part of you dictate your food choices.

- Seeing what your body will choose if you let it.

- Becoming more open and intuitive in other areas of your life.

- Deepening your connection to yourself and learning to trust your innate wisdom more deeply.

Adopting the Habits of an Intuitive Eater

- Before you go to eat your next meal or snack ask, 'What does my body really want right now?' and listen for the answer.

- Believe and intend that your body will make the best food choices possible for you.

- Be open to surprise information or 'cravings'.

- Allow your body to direct you to new foods when you next go shopping or foraging.

- Surrender to your intuition but still engage your brain!

Integrating with Other Types

Integrated with the Functional Eater

The Intuitive Eater and the Functional Eater are already very similar in so many ways: they both love food to be quick, clean and easy to eat/prepare; they both like simple, sometimes plain foods, and they both like to eat what they enjoy and are very straightforward about it. Also, both types rarely have any types of hang-ups about food or eating, and they tend not to eat unless they are hungry (except when mixed with those types who eat even when they're not), so they are naturally very compatible.

That said, it usually only pays the Intuitive Eater to integrate with the Functional Eater when they've somehow started to make their food choices overcomplicated, which can lead to a lack of connection. When this happens, using the Functional Eater's simple approach to food can bring the Intuitive Eater back to wholeness and balance.

Integrated with the Sensual Eater

The Intuitive Eater and the Sensual Eater are both 'feeling' types who thrive on having a heightened experience around food. Integrating with the Sensual Eater can be beneficial if the Intuitive Eater is looking to enjoy and appreciate eating and food even more, and/or to move into trying new foods or different ways with foods, which may take them into an even deeper experience and relationship with what they consume. That aside, for the Intuitive Eater who is already in a really good place with their eating, it would be considered a regression rather than progression to integrate with the Sensual Eater because the Sensual Eater is driven by pleasure rather than instinct. If the Intuitive Eater is already experiencing enough pleasure in their diet then there is very little value to be gained here via this integration.

Integrated with the Intellectual Eater

The Intellectual Eater can be the perfect integration for the Intuitive Eater, especially the one who has never taken the time to understand food and nutrition in any great detail. As aware and sensitive as the Intuitive Eater may be, without an equally strong intellectual knowledge about *what* they are eating and what suits them best, they run the risk of moving through life in partial darkness about whether what they are eating is truly best for them or not. Once this particular integration has taken place, the Intuitive Eater can evolve even more fully and move forward with greater confidence than ever before.

Integrated with the Emotional Eater

The Intuitive Eater has no need to integrate with the Emotional Eater, and nothing can be gained from it, that is unless they opt to become an Emotional Eater purely for the experience and awareness of it, and what that can bring. This would be helpful if the Intuitive Eater feels as if they need some kind of inner breakthrough and chooses to use food as a way of flagging up problem areas, but it would have to be a controlled experiment, otherwise it could lead to a long-term habit.

Integrated with the Focused Eater

Every type can benefit from integrating with the Focused Eater, and in this case, for the Intuitive Eater specifically, it's the highest integration of all. Because the Intuitive Eater is already pretty evolved, bringing the influence of the Focused Eater into the mix enables them to create one or more specific goals and reach them in a way that feels good. For the Intuitive Eater this brings a valuable sense of achievement, because sometimes their eating can verge on feeling aimless. It also enables them to create some more healthy boundaries around what they do and don't eat, just in case their 'intuitive' eating starts to become mindless.

Integrated with the Conscious Eater

Integrating with the Conscious Eater is usually not at all difficult for the Intuitive Eater because both types are on a very similar wavelength already, where they feel their way to their decisions. Where the Conscious Eater does this usually via their mind and emotions, the Intuitive Eater does it via their body. This means that for the Intuitive Eater, integrating with the Conscious Eater can feel like rounding out an already conscious equation into one that feels even more sound and holistic still. This is a very peaceful combination.

Integrated with the Experimental Eater

It's particularly useful to the Intuitive Eater to integrate with the Experimental Eater when they are bored with the foods they keep choosing, are looking to reinvent themselves, and/or feel ready to cast their culinary net further afield. Even though the Intuitive Eater usually does a great job of staying in balance with their diet, periodically there can come times when they feel like shaking things up or following a new philosophy of eating. At times like these they will naturally move towards integration with the Experimental Eater in order to explore new terrain in a way that is exciting to them.

Integrated with the Confused Eater

While the Intuitive Eater is all about clarity, the Confused Eater is in a very different place that is of no use to the Intuitive Eater at all – that is, unless, as with the Emotional Eater integration, it is temporary and for a specific purpose. This type of situation might arise when the Intuitive Eater is opening up to new ideas and thoughts around food and is prepared to go back to basics in a bid to upgrade their approach to food. In this instance, allowing a certain amount of confusion/uncertainty would be the natural evolution of things as the Intuitive Eater prepares to enter a whole new world of experience and possibility.

Integrated with the Social Eater

Becoming more of a Social Eater is not a big problem for the Intuitive Eater, who typically eats from a diverse range of foods anyway. In fact, this integration can be a very fun one, creating something of an 'edge' for the Intuitive Eater as they prepare to take on the challenge of being intuitive from a printed menu rather than a real live fridge. Although an Intuitive Eater's preference would be to choose foods fresh from their own home or local store, what they can appreciate about integrating with the Social Eater is the opportunity to discover new foods and new approaches to food which will potentially add more options and ideas to future meal choices.

The Conscious Evolution of the Intuitive Eater

The Intuitive Eater is primarily tuned in to their body, heart and soul.

- **In its weakest expression:** can struggle to discern true intuition from something else entirely and end up creating health issues.

- **In its highest expression:** you are finely tuned in to your body and self in a way that is inspiring, and you feel confident and happy that you are eating day to day, moment to moment in the way that is perfect for you.

The ultimate evolution for the Intuitive Eater is to make sure that they are not in denial of any aspect of themselves by embodying the following Eater Types: Sensual + Intellectual + Conscious + Focused.

When the Intuitive Eater does this they create the experience of:

- loving the food they eat
- knowing that what they are eating is great for them
- feeling genuinely happy with their food choices from an ethical standpoint
- having some kind of 'point' to what they are eating so it doesn't run the risk of becoming too random (and, ultimately, unhelpful).

See pages 253–55 for some great food ideas for the healthy Intuitive Eater.

SIGNATURE DISH FOR THE INTUITIVE EATER

almond-banana milk

This recipe is clean-tasting, delicious and filling. It works perfectly for the Intuitive Eater because it's made from pure ingredients, is easily digested and is also highly nutritious and satisfying on every level.

Serves   1–2

Equipment   Blender and nut milk bag/fine sieve/strainer

Ingredients   1 cup almonds OR 1 tbsp raw almond butter

3 cups pure water

1 large banana or 2 small–medium bananas

2–4 medjool dates (to your taste)

Directions

- Place the almonds and water in a blender and blend until all the almonds are broken up.
- If you use whole almonds and not almond butter (and therefore need to strain the milk), use a nut milk bag or very fine sieve to strain the mixture so that you separate the almond skin from the milk. When you've done this, pour the clean nut milk into your clean blender jug.
- Add your banana/s to the almond milk and blend until well combined.
- Taste-test the milk. If it's not sweet enough, add some dates and blend again.
- Repeat until you find your perfect combination.

KAREN'S TIPS

This drink is great for breakfast, as a snack or as a light supper. This is best drunk right away, otherwise the banana will separate out and go slightly brown.

The almond milk alone makes an excellent base for any smoothie.

THE CONSCIOUS EATER 🍎

The Conscious Eater operates from what they would consider to be their heart and/or soul. Their food, and usually all other life choices, are generated by what they believe to be the highest or most pure path – the kindest one – and they find a way of making it work for this very reason.

Conscious Eaters typically see themselves as being in service to their path rather than the other way around. The food that they eat is very much viewed as an illustration and demonstration of their depth of spirituality and consciousness, and they believe in it very passionately. Taken to the extreme, the Conscious Eater dreams of a world where everything we eat is as local, clean, nutritious and cruelty-free as possible, and all unnecessary greed, starvation, planetary pollution and suffering is a thing of the past.

The Conscious Eater's view –

- on food: 'Nourishing'

- on eating: 'Sacred'

- on self-catering: 'Perfect'

- on takeaways: 'Never'

- on being personally catered for: 'OK'

- on eating out: 'Unnecessary'

- on changing their diet: 'If it's a higher and healthier path for all concerned, then take me to it.'

The Conscious Eater and Pleasure

Conscious Eaters love it when…

- they feel they have found their way or, even better, the 'ultimate' way. Conscious Eaters are driven by their desire to be the best they can be – but with ethics. There are always conditions attached with the Conscious Eater (a very good thing) and so they are much more discerning than any other Eater Type. This discernment and their high moral and spiritual standards can lead them to a very clean, pure and ethical path very quickly. Once they find one, they feel truly at peace with themselves, and when they learn about something even better, just watch the smile of gratitude and excitement wash over their face!

- **they take the higher ground.** Conscious Eaters are as human as the next person and so they are not immune to the addictions and temptations of this world. As 'real' as that may be, and because of this, Conscious Eaters pride themselves on their ability to rise above the mainstream and to make choices that come from a higher, more evolved place within. Of course, being face-to-face with an old 'friend' or addiction and choosing the better choice is a sure-fire recipe for feeling wonderful about themselves.

- **they have a positive influence on someone else.** Conscious Eaters can get very passionate about their cause – whatever shape or form that may take. Some are big on eating locally, others on organics, others on going veggie or vegan, or treating animals more humanely; these are just a selection of the causes which the Conscious Eater is likely to champion. In any case, nothing makes the Conscious Eater feel more proud or valid in their beliefs than having someone agree with them to the extent that they change their own life. Although Conscious Eaters would love for the whole world to change overnight, for now they can feel happy about changing the planet one life at a time.

The Conscious Eater's idea of heaven: 'Living on a planet where everything we eat is grown, made and prepared with love and nothing suffers or dies unnecessarily for our appetite.'

The Conscious Eater and Pain

Conscious Eaters struggle when…

- **their 'ideal diet' doesn't yield ideal results.** The risk that Conscious Eaters tend to run is that, in their bid to eat the cleanest, healthiest and purest diet, they can sometimes take things too far, miss out key nutrients or, worse, starve their body in their efforts to do things 'right'. This can be avoided by staying grounded, paying attention to what works and looking for the happy ground where all the boxes can be ticked.

- **they make a food choice that goes against their moral grain.** Now and again there may be times when Conscious Eaters aren't able to eat the way they want to eat due to circumstance – or they simply have a rebellious moment. When this happens, depending on their attitude and beliefs, it can cause anything from minor discord to full-on panic. The solution here is to be really clear on what is and isn't OK and then to be prepared for every situation.

- **they witness cruelty, inconsiderateness or unconsciousness in others.** Nothing pains the Conscious Eater more than to witness pain, pollution, suffering or anything they perceive as negative happening at the hands of their fellow (wo)man. Quite simply, they have invested so much time and energy into becoming a higher version of themselves that they feel frustrated when others haven't got on the same boat at the same time, headed for the same destination.

The Conscious Eater's idea of hell: 'Living in a world where the land is abused, animals are slaughtered, crops are poisoned and all sense of sacredness, respect and compassion are gone.'

If This Is You

If you are a Conscious Eater, or if this fits part of your Eater Type profile, bookmark this page for a second and turn to Chapter 2 (page 126), where there are three short but revealing questions for you to consider. These will help you get more in touch with how being a Conscious Eater has both worked for you *and* caused you issues. You don't have to do anything with this information just yet, but please don't skip it; it is vital. Take this opportunity to reflect on things; you may well have one or two 'Aha!' moments that could be of tremendous value to you. Once you've done that, come back to this page and keep reading.

. . . .

Case Study: Greg, 35, Glasgow

Greg began his work with me by explaining that he had been a vegan for 12 years and was very happy with his lifestyle choice. Staying vegan was important to him, so Greg didn't want to make any changes there. Aside from that, he felt well, looked healthy and had taken the time to make sure he had created a well-balanced, highly nutritious diet so he could sustain his lifestyle without issue. However, in spite of feeling good about what and how he was eating, he felt that something important was missing. This was what he had come to me to explore.

As I listened to him I could tell that, despite being a Conscious Eater, Greg had slipped into an unconsciousness around his own needs as an individual. Upon further discussion, it became clear that in his bid to 'do the right thing' with his diet and his passion for animal welfare, he had slowly but surely neglected his *own* emotional needs – it was time to take care of himself.

I suggested to Greg that perhaps the missing ingredients were 'joy' and 'self-love' in his diet. Absolutely I could see how eating in accordance with his beliefs and ethics made him happy and helped him to maintain a strong sense of integrity, but as it was now a regular, fixed part of his way of being, and had been for over a decade; the original joy at taking this stand had simply become part of his identity and was no longer fresh or exciting for him.

Realizing the truth of this, Greg agreed that this felt like the 'hot spot' he was looking for in our work together. And so it was that we started brainstorming and discussing what would get him excited again about food, eating and extending to himself the same loving, considerate and thoughtful standards as he did to his animal friends.

This question fascinated him and excited him at the same time. In all his years of caring and thinking about animals and aligning his diet with compassion, he had never once held himself and his own value up to the same degree – *and he finally got that this was just as important.*

During our work together we looked at a multitude of ways that Greg could bring more joy and self-love into his diet – for him and him alone – while staying on his Conscious Eater path. The quiz had revealed that, while most of his answers related to the Conscious Eater, he also found himself wishing that he was more of a Social Eater as he missed the companionship that he once had enjoyed through social gatherings before he became vegan. It seemed like a great idea to work with this so, among other things, Greg took the time to find and proactively connect with vegan groups and networks and to attend meals out and other social events to nourish that part of himself again. This in and of itself made a huge difference, but also integrating with the Experimental Eater brought him the energy and impetus to try new and different foods and to inject more of his own desires and fun into his diet.

In the time that we worked together Greg literally became a new man. Without compromising his vegan ethics one bit, he changed from a stay-at-home philosopher to the life and soul of the party. He had found his tribe, was experimenting with exciting new foods and recipes and, most important of all, was finally treating himself with the level of love, respect and humility that he well and truly deserves.

The Benefits of Being a Conscious Eater

- Allows you to integrate your ethics or beliefs with your eating habits.

- Makes it possible to feel in alignment with every area of your life.

- Great for you if you are passionate about making the world a better place.

- You can feel really good about what you're eating on a spiritual level.

- Applying a moral or ethical code to your food choices could help you where you need it.

Adopting the Habits of a Conscious Eater

- Get clear on what your ethical or moral code is, exactly.

- Make a list of the now 'taboo' foods and drinks and remove them from your diet.

- See if your body agrees with your new way of eating – it may or may not.

- Use your meal times as opportunities for conscious connection to the self and the divine.

- Give thanks for everything you have to eat and drink and bless it.

Integrating with Other Types

Integrated with the Functional Eater

The Functional Eater is an especially good integration for the Conscious Eater who could benefit from keeping things simple, such as one carrying excess weight or who would like to simplify their life and diet. For the Conscious Eater who has an especially busy mind around their reasons for being conscious, keeping the actual eating part simple can help offset the mental stress with a physical ease that can be very beneficial. This integration would not be so positive, however, if the Conscious Eater didn't feel truly abundant in their choices. If they were to integrate with the Functional Eater they might just tip over the edge into feeling as if their existence had become too stark or restricted in some way.

Integrated with the Sensual Eater

Becoming more of a Sensual Eater is a good strategy for the Conscious Eater who is starting to feel any sense of martyrdom as a result of their conscious choices. By becoming more sensual and indulgent around their food they can instead start to feel as if their ethical concerns have taken them to a more vibrant, interesting place. This will help them feel even more positive about every choice they make because of where these choices lead them.

Integrated with the Intellectual Eater

Input from the Intellectual Eater can be the perfect tonic for the Conscious Eater who has become blinkered in their thinking/feeling around a well-balanced diet. Sometimes Conscious Eaters can restrict their diet considerably in their bid to eat (or not eat) in a particular way, so integrating with the Intellectual Eater will ensure that they stay mindful of keeping or becoming healthy, so that they can confidently uphold their philosophy without being damaged along the way.

Integrated with the Emotional Eater

Blending the Conscious Eater with the Emotional Eater would not be the greatest integration, because often the Conscious Eater is already emotional enough around food owing to their very strong opinions and beliefs. If this integration *were* to occur, it could lead to a lot of additional, unnecessary tension and drama around food, which could easily be avoided by integrating with a different type instead.

The Conscious Eater will find a lot more joy in choosing a type that helps them feel good about what they're doing rather than focusing on more of what they *don't* want, which is what the Conscious Eater is ultimately trying to move away from.

Integrated with the Focused Eater

A Conscious Eater who chooses to integrate with the Focused Eater can create a very interesting life and experience indeed. By focusing on achieving specific goals or aims, the Conscious Eater can channel all their passion, drive and focus into something that makes a positive difference in a way that is truly fulfilling to them and, potentially, to many other people, too. For the Conscious Eater who already cares deeply for other beings, this can feel like the ultimate win–win, something that is very attractive to them and has the potential to change the face of the planet for the better.

Integrated with the Intuitive Eater

These two types have one major thing in common: a strong sense of spirituality and/or connection to their food and, most likely, to everything else around them. For this reason, integrating the Conscious Eater with the Intuitive Eater can be a joyful, easy and spiritually powerful union, where the Conscious Eater gets to indulge even more fully in surrendering to other more 'awake' parts of themselves and seeing where this takes them.

On one level this is a great integration to make. On another, the Conscious Eater needs to remain mindful that adding another type to bring common sense and groundedness to the mix would be a wise thing to do, so that they keep their feet on the ground and stay or become as fit, strong and healthy as they desire.

Integrated with the Experimental Eater

Normally the Conscious Eater sees their food path as narrowing rather than broadening when they start to eschew certain types of foods from their diet in order to become conscious. By integrating with the Experimental Eater they have the opportunity to reverse this trend and instead to open up to more diverse ways of eating, to new foods, to alternative foods that may taste, look or feel similar to those they've given up but that are issue-free. This is an integration that would probably last just a short while in order to serve its purpose, however, as Experimental Eaters usually do not concern themselves with any of the issues that Conscious Eaters are so passionate about.

Integrated with the Confused Eater

A Conscious Eater may automatically integrate with the Confused Eater when they start to doubt something about their criteria/choices at any stage of their food journey. When this happens, the relationship can go one of two ways: either the Conscious Eater starts to doubt or question everything that they've come to believe (and go through all the emotional and intellectual turbulence that this doubt may bring), or they use the inner conversations instigated by the integration to come out the other side even stronger. Consequently, this particular integration is recommended only for those who are ready to go through that intellectual baptism of fire.

Integrated with the Social Eater

Most Conscious Eaters naturally struggle with the thought of becoming a Social Eater. Not surprising, given that Social Eaters are not renowned for their A1 sense of ethics. As a result, the thought of integrating with the Social Eater is not necessarily one that thrills the Conscious Eater, although there are some powerful positives that can come about as a result. First of all, the Conscious Eater has an opportunity, at every social venue, to make a difference. By asking for what they want, they get to vote with their wallet. Second, as there are now some fantastic ethical and sustainable food establishments around, all the great things that go with that are waiting to be enjoyed – and supported, so that they can stay in business and thrive. For any Conscious Eater who would like to make a difference to food/eating in the mainstream, this is an integration that could certainly position them for creating some social changes that will have an even bigger impact than their individual private choices.

The Conscious Evolution of the Conscious Eater

The Conscious Eater is primarily tuned in to their heart and soul.

- **In its weakest expression:** can ignore the body and intellect completely and encounter deficiencies (through limiting their food groups) that do their physical body harm.

- **In its highest expression:** you eat a wide diversity of high-quality foods which you feel great about, your physical body is thriving and, as a result of your choices, you feel spiritually connected to yourself, the planet and the universe.

The ultimate evolution for the Conscious Eater is to make sure that they create or maintain a truly healthy whole-person balance by embodying the following Eater Types: Sensual + Intellectual + Intuitive + Focused.

When the Conscious Eater does this they create the experience of:

- loving the food they eat
- knowing that what they are eating is great for them
- being more tuned in to their body and what *it* wants
- reaching/maintaining their personal goals, whatever these may be.

See pages 253–55 for some great food ideas for the healthy Conscious Eater.

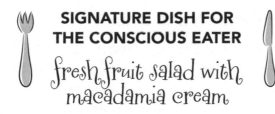

SIGNATURE DISH FOR THE CONSCIOUS EATER

fresh fruit salad with macadamia cream

Perfect for planet-friendly Conscious Eaters, a fresh fruit salad is one of the best meals on Earth. And when it's topped with this macadamia cream, it's *heaven* on Earth. This is a fabulously refreshing and sustaining meal at any time of day.

Serves   1–2

Equipment Blender or hand blender

Ingredients Fruits of choice

One handful raw macadamia nuts

Juice of half an orange (or a whole one, depending on juiciness)

2–4 large medjool dates (or 4–8 smaller soaked ones)

Small piece of vanilla bean (optional)

Directions

- Prepare your fruit salad using a wide range of fresh juicy fruits of your choice. A good mixture might be: banana, orange, apple, strawberries, nectarines and blueberries.

- Next, make your topping by blending all the other ingredients together until a thick, creamy mixture is created.

- Taste-test before using and add more of whatever you need.

- Serve your fruit salad and top with a good healthy serving of the deliciously dreamy macadamia cream.

KAREN'S TIPS

This recipe will keep for about two to three days in the fridge. Great for topping breakfasts to make something a bit more sustaining, and you can also add a tablespoon or two to your next fruit smoothie.

THE EXPERIMENTAL EATER 🍎

Experimental Eaters like to… experiment! They see life as a vast smorgasbord of adventure and possibility, and if something exists then it must be there to be experienced, right? Experimental Eaters are never happier than when they are trying something new, just so they can tick something else off a never-ending list, plus they get to tell the tale! They're usually very sociable and gregarious types and often combine their experimental tendencies with socializing so that they can get even more mileage out of the experience.

For the Experimental Eater, eating is all about diversity, abundance and unlimited possibilities.

The Experimental Eater's view –

- on food: 'Fascinating'

- on eating: 'Gratifying'

- on self-catering: 'OK-ish'

- on takeaways: 'So-so'

- on being personally catered for: 'Nice'

- on eating out: 'Yay!'

- on changing their diet: 'If I get introduced to new foods that I love, then I'm up for anything.'

The Experimental Eater and Pleasure

Experimental Eaters love it when…

- **they discover a food or ingredient that they've never had before.** Experimental Eaters love trying new things – and the more exotic or unusual, the better. For them, everything about food means trying something new or enjoying old favourites in a new and interesting way.

- **they travel and get to experience different cultures' food-related specialities, rituals and traditions.** Experimental Eaters love to try foods from all around the world, for so many different reasons. Even if they aren't great travellers themselves, they will never pass up an invite to visit an obscure or unusual restaurant to try new foods and approaches to food and to learn more about the diversity of the world.

- **something that they share with others about a food experience creates a stir or starts a conversation.** Experimental Eaters are usually in it for themselves, but they certainly aren't averse to causing a stir or inspiring a conversation about the contents of their fridge or what bizarre choice they've just made from the restaurant menu. Some Experimental Eaters make choices that could be considered shocking to others, but to them it's just another day at the table.

The Experimental Eater's idea of heaven: 'Travelling around the globe (or a city) trying every country's native dish and enjoying all their culinary secrets.'

The Experimental Eater and Pain

Experimental Eaters struggle when...

- **their food gets plain or lacks interest or diversity.** Experimental Eaters thrive on diversity because there are so many foods in the world waiting to be tried – why waste another day eating the 'same old, same old'?

- **they get stuck in a food rut.** As with anyone who gets caught in a busy daily routine and doesn't have time to play with food, the Experimental Eater is always open to the risk of getting stuck in a food rut the same as anyone else. When this happens, a big night out or weekend away inevitably ensues – anything to break the mould and get something different pumping round the veins!

- **they go on a 'health-kick' and they get bored, bored, bored.** Experimental Eaters who want to get healthy can struggle massively when they try to follow a stereotypical diet plan. In order for them to succeed they need to make a point of bringing in the weird, wonderful, spicy, decadent or whatever else floats their boat to create a menu plan that still feels as exciting and expansive as any other.

The Experimental Eater's idea of hell: 'Having to eat the same (plain) food over and over again – and, even worse, eating it by myself.'

If This Is You

If you are an Experimental Eater, or if this fits part of your Eater Type profile, bookmark this page for a second and turn to Chapter 2 (page 126), where you'll find three short (but revealing!) questions I'd like you to have a think about. These will help you get more in touch with how being an Experimental Eater has worked for you *and* caused issues. You don't have to do anything with this information just yet, but don't skip it; it is vital. Take this opportunity to reflect on things; you may well have one or two 'Aha!' moments that could be of tremendous value to you. Once you've done that, come back to this page and keep reading.

. . . .

Case Study: Patrick, 27, Belgium

As an Experimental Eater and a high-flying international executive on a very high salary, Patrick had always taken great pleasure in eating out at exclusive and unusual restaurants around the world, as part of his unique and lavish lifestyle. In fact, it was one of the pleasures in life that he truly lived for. Nothing pleased Patrick more than to discover a new food or drink that got his taste-buds tingling – a pleasure further instigated by the Sensual Eater in his Eater Type profile, which was almost just as dominant.

Apart from some minor health concerns and a slightly rotund midriff, there was no real reason for Patrick to stop or question his excessive lifestyle until the unexpected happened – redundancy.

It was then that he had to stop, think and make a plan for how he was going to move forward in life *and* find a way to satiate the Experimental and Sensual Eaters within.

After getting clear on specific numbers so we knew exactly what he *could* spend on food a month, and finding out more about his health issues so we could address those as well, I shared with Patrick information about the different Eater Types and, in the spirit of play and adventure, asked him to choose another one or two that he felt he could have some fun with during this time, so that he didn't migrate towards focusing on 'lack'. This way he could, instead, move into a different place with his experience, and effectively drink from a new source of diversity and abundance. He loved this idea – especially as it was already clear that for him to feel truly alive and prosperous he was not going to be able to rely solely on fine foods or money anymore, especially with the international jet-setting out of the equation.

Patrick decided that the Social Eater and the Conscious Eater were the two Eater Types that he'd like to experiment with. At first I was surprised – after all, this was a young man who seemed completely uninterested in anything 'conscious' at all. However, he explained that in spite of his indulgent past, the redundancy had been a wake-up call on more than just a financial level, and he wanted to use this time and his work with me to experiment with another *completely different* way of viewing and interacting with food – 'just to see'.

I agreed that this was a brilliant idea, especially perfect for an Experimental Eater, and so it was that we set about creating a brand new life and lifestyle for him. Instead of choosing dishes from expensive restaurant menus, Patrick started scoping out the finest delis and health food stores.

Instead of paying for a group of friends to eat out at the swankiest eatery in town, he learned how to cook and prepare healthy, ingenious dishes and became quite the chef and 'host with the most' within a few short months. And, instead of getting excited about trying an exotic or fancy restaurant, his enthusiasm gravitated towards creating 'mocktails' out of healthy fresh juices, wild herbs and liquid superfoods!

As you can imagine, our time together was progressive, inspiring and rewarding. To this day I still marvel at how clever and imaginative Experimental Eaters can be when they need to be, and Patrick was certainly no exception.

The Benefits of Being an Experimental Eater

- Learning to try new things if you are used to playing safe with food.

- Shaking things up a bit if you're bored with your diet.

- Creating new recipes with new foods or ingredients.

- Learning that healthy eating has way more to offer than you know.

- Becoming ready to spread your wings in other areas of your life.

Adopting the Habits of an Experimental Eater

- Set a project for yourself that means you must expand your horizons.

- Make a point of trying one new food a week.

- Go shopping for food where you've never been before.

- Eat at a new raw restaurant or juice bar and try something new.

- Attend a raw food class and expand your repertoire.

Integrating with Other Types

Integrated with the Functional Eater

Perhaps not the best integration for the Experimental Eater, the Functional Eater is pretty middle-of-the-road when it comes to food and eating, and is not known for having extravagant tastes or habits – far from it. Where this integration could be useful, however, is if the Experimental Eater in question has gone experimental to the max and needs a little toning down and/or wants to simplify things. In either case, integrating with the Functional Eater would certainly take care of this and lead to a more sedate relationship with food – if that's what's required.

Integrated with the Sensual Eater

When these two types integrate it's a potent combination indeed. Both types are renowned for their indulgent tendencies and exploratory nature around food. Both types love to adventure internally and externally with food and see where it takes them. So, when the Experimental Eater chooses to integrate with the Sensual Eater it's going to be because they want to go 'double-deep' into their experience and enjoy greater intimacy with their food. For the Experimental Eater who wants to explore the depths of eating for pleasure and self-gratification, this is the most powerful integration imaginable; however, for the Experimental Eater who suffers from excess weight, food addiction or any other negative eating-related conditions, it would be a recipe for disaster.

Integrated with the Intellectual Eater

Any Experimental Eater who wants to know more about where their food comes from, how it is made and whether it's good for them would benefit greatly from integrating with the Intellectual Eater. The level-headedness and fact-finding tendencies of the Intellectual Eater will brilliantly complement the 'gay abandon' of the Experimental Eater, who, ordinarily, doesn't tend to care about any of the above – unless it translates into a fascinating fact that they can impress an audience with, of course. The other big plus of this particular integration is that the mindfulness of the Intellectual Eater will ensure that the Experimental Eater doesn't trade experience for health. This is an especially big deal for this type, as their fascination and love affair with food can often have a well-being price tag on it that is way more expensive than the restaurant bills they've racked up.

Integrated with the Emotional Eater

Integrating with the Emotional Eater makes no sense whatsoever for the Experimental Eater. There is nothing that they can gain here that would be of any significant value to them, especially as they don't generally have any kind of mastery around food, so wouldn't have a safety net to fall back on. If they did choose to do this, be it consciously or unconsciously, what would be likely to ensue is a very messy-looking lifestyle and very possibly a lot of 'whole person' damage. Not recommended!

Integrated with the Focused Eater

If they feel they want to move to another level in their food experience, then the Experimental Eater should call on the Focused Eater for the fast-track to the top. With its laser-like focus and drive to reach specific goals, the Focused Eater can bring so much value and stability to the Experimental Eater's diet. Yes, it would call for a level of control which the Experimental Eater may never have demonstrated before, but as Experimental Eaters are usually highly intelligent and up for a challenge they could actually come to love the stretch this offers, as it indulges the side of them that likes to 'eat and see what happens'. For this experience, there surely cannot be a more helpful or fascinating combination.

Integrated with the Intuitive Eater

At first glance you might think these two types could never work well together or integrate easily, as one is pleasure driven and the other much more conscious, but actually the influence of the Intuitive Eater can be extremely beneficial for the Experimental Eater, and very easy to integrate when the motives align. In this case, for this to happen joyfully the Experimental Eater would need to be ready to become more health conscious and prepared to establish a deeper and more holistic relationship with themselves. This would need to be the case because, once they started listening to their body in true Intuitive Eater style, what would very likely be revealed to them would be that not everything they like to eat actually does them good. For anyone, letting go of unhelpful foods means they need to be ready to move to a higher internal terrain. For the Experimental Eater, integrating with the Intuitive Eater would be one of the best choices they could possibly make to get them to that special place.

Integrated with the Conscious Eater

If the Experimental Eater is looking for personal evolution, then one of the biggest areas for improvement is going to concern becoming more conscious around what they eat and why. In this case, integrating with the Conscious Eater is going to be the perfect solution. Adopting the habits of the Conscious Eater can help the Experimental Eater to think beyond themselves and consider the ethical, environmental and ecological impact of what they're eating. This will make all the difference: the Experimental Eater will find a new, more spiritual depth to their journey with food, which they may never have experienced before. From this place they have the opportunity to find that wonderful place where head, heart, body and taste-buds are all feeling happy and aligned.

Integrated with the Confused Eater

It's highly unlikely that the Experimental Eater will ever get intertwined with the Confused Eater. The only way this could or would happen is if an Experimental Eater were to decide they wanted to eat more healthily or pursue a certain food 'path' and started feeling confused or overwhelmed along the way. The good news is that, with Experimental Eaters being the smart cookies they are, this would likely only be a short-term sojourn. Within a matter of days it's highly likely that they'd find their way and be off and running with confidence and their own new brand of experimentation.

Integrated with the Social Eater

It's not a big ask to have the Experimental Eater and Social Eater combine. Both love to try new things, and neither is much bothered by what the menu brings, so long as it's tasty, interesting and gives them something to talk about and get excited about. For this reason, for the Experimental Eater who wants to become even more of a socialite this is the integration to go for. When these two get together, many hours of fun, food and frivolity await.

The Conscious Evolution of the Experimental Eater

The Experimental Eater is primarily tuned in to their mind (and taste-buds!).

- **In its weakest expression:** consumes literally anything that doesn't run away, and becomes gluttonous, selfish and constantly craving.

- **In its highest expression:** you adore pursuing new foods and tastes with a passion and you do it with a reverence and genuine sense of gratitude and appreciation that is touching.

The ultimate evolution for the Experimental Eater is to move out of eating purely for the experience and evolve into embodying the following Eater Types: Sensual + Intellectual + Conscious + Intuitive + Focused.

When the Experimental Eater does this they create the experience of:

- loving the food they eat
- knowing that what they are eating is great for them
- feeling genuinely happy with their food choices from an ethical standpoint
- being more tuned in to their body and what *it* wants
- reaching/maintaining their personal health/body goals, whatever these may be.

See pages 253–55 for some great food ideas for the healthy Experimental Eater.

SIGNATURE DISH FOR THE EXPERIMENTAL EATER

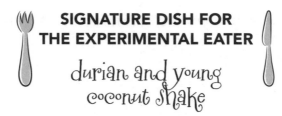

durian and young coconut shake

Take two of the world's finest natural creations – durian is known in southeast Asia as 'the king of fruits' – and whizz them in a blender: the Experimental Eater doesn't just get exotic and unusual, but also a super-healthy and tasty meal-in-a-drink to boot.

Serves   1–2

Equipment   Blender

Ingredients   One young coconut

Two small segments of durian flesh

Directions

- Open your young coconut using a sharp knife or cleaver so that the top pops off and the flesh and 'water' are exposed.

- Pour out the coconut water into a blender. Scoop out the flesh using a spoon and add to the blender.

- Pit the durian flesh and add the flesh, minus stones, to the blender in small pieces.

- Blend everything together until a lovely thick shake is created.

KAREN'S TIP

Blend with a little ice for an even more chilled and exotic version.

THE CONFUSED EATER 🍏

The Confused Eater is generally not a happy bunny when it comes to food. They desperately want to be happy (or say they do!) but spend a good portion of their life and life-force energy wondering what they should be eating and if they could be doing better, or worrying about what they have eaten and whether it was the best choice after all.

The main issue for the Confused Eater is their reluctance to tune in to their own wisdom; this may well play out in other areas of their life, with equally frustrating and debilitating consequences. For the Confused Eater the world of food and eating is a minefield, and one that they keep trying to navigate even when it stops being fun.

The Confused Eater's view –

- on food: 'Confusing'

- on eating: 'Frustrating'

- on self-catering: 'Fine'

- on takeaways: 'Ugh'

- on being personally catered for: 'Super'

- on eating out: 'OK...'

- on changing their diet: 'If I'm told exactly what to eat and specifically why it's good for me, then I'll do it – so long as it makes sense to me.'

The Confused Eater and Pleasure

Confused Eaters love it when...

- **they gain some clarity about some aspect of food or eating that's been bothering them.** Confused Eaters are always open to new information because, like the Intellectual Eater, they're always looking for the 'right way' to eat. So when they obtain a piece of information that sounds or feels good to them, they're all over it, as if someone has just thrown them a life raft.

- **they read a book that makes complete sense.** Confused Eaters generally do love to read health books and articles in their search for the answers that they're seeking. Periodically they will come across a book that feels so perfect and sounds like the ultimate way. When this happens it's champagne-on-ice time – but only if the author would allow it, of course…

- **they feel as if they have finally 'got it'.** When this day arrives it's a whole lifetime of birthdays all wrapped up in one! If and when this happens, the Confused Eater gets to 'graduate' to the next level, finally moving out of confusion and into a place of peace, clarity and positivity. Eureka!

The Confused Eater's idea of heaven: 'Being handed a book entitled Every Question You've Ever Had About Food Answered.*'*

The Confused Eater and Pain

Confused Eaters struggle when…

- **they try something different and it doesn't work.** Confused Eaters are certainly game when it comes to making changes to their diet, but unfortunately these changes have a tendency to not always work out quite the way they had hoped. This is usually because the terrain on which the changes are being made is not as sound as it could be. Like the Emotional Eater, the Confused Eater's true path to success lies through mastery of the inside rather than anything spectacular landing in their lap from the outside. This gets to happen later.

- **they start to question something they truly believed.** A lot of stock is put in 'things that work' when a Confused

Eater finds them. Like a jigsaw puzzle that must be pieced together, Confused Eaters collect data in their quest to get it all figured out. So when one of the puzzle pieces starts to crumble and fall, it's a very sad day indeed. When this happens, they have no other choice but to replace that particular puzzle piece, and so the journey continues.

- **they attend a lecture or read a book that turns everything on its head.** This scenario happens frequently with the Confused Eater, as there are infinite ideas about what we should eat and why. The fact of the matter is, this is never going to change. Everyone in life has to figure out 'their' way, and the sooner the Confused Eater steps into a more personalized and holistic approach to eating, the sooner their pain, confusion and frustration will come to a long-awaited end.

The Confused Eater's idea of hell: 'Being in a lecture hall with 20 different nutritionists who dramatically disagree with one another.'

If This Is You

If you are a Confused Eater, or if this fits part of your Eater Type profile, bookmark this page for a second and turn to Chapter 2 (page 126), where there are three short (but revealing!) questions I'd like you to consider. These will help you get more in touch with how being a Confused Eater has worked for you *and* caused issues. You don't have to do anything with this information just yet, but don't skip it; it is vital. Take this opportunity to reflect on things; you may well have one or two 'Aha!' moments that could be of tremendous value to you. Once you've done that, come back to this page and keep reading.

Case Study: Marilyn, 30, Belfast

As Marilyn and I spoke for the first time, I did not need the quiz to confirm for me that Marilyn was a truly Confused Eater. Sharing with me her frustration and desperation about what and what not to eat, I felt genuine compassion for her plight, and I knew I could help her – if only she could get clear on what exactly it was that she wanted!

We explored many options: weight loss? ('Nope.') Increased energy? ('Not really...') Health issues? ('No problem there.') Clarity? ('Obviously, but there's more to it than that...')

As I ran through the list of different health-related options we could work with and focus on in order to create the perfect plan for her, nothing was really striking a chord with Marilyn – until I asked, 'So why are you really here?'

It was then that she shared with me that she wasn't just confused about what to eat, but also about who she was, what she wanted and where she was going in her life. Bottom line: she was flat out confused about just about everything.

It's not uncommon for Confused Eaters to be confused in other areas of their life, just as it's not uncommon for Focused Eaters to be focused, Sensual Eaters to be sensual, and so on. In fact, as the saying goes, 'How we do something is how we do everything' – in my experience, this tends to be true.

And so I decided, especially after hearing the extent to which this was a theme of her life, that, rather than try and push for anything concrete from Marilyn, we would try the 'lie back and see' approach.

I explained to Marilyn that this approach basically meant she could eat whatever she wanted, but that if we were to work together there would be just one simple condition: she would keep a detailed record of her physical, emotional and mental responses to every food and drink choice that she made.

As this sounded easy enough to do and gave her a high degree of focus without any additional 'what do I eat?'

pressure, it was clear to us both that this was definitely the way to go.

For the next 10 days Marilyn kept her food diary, as agreed. Apart from a couple of days where she lost sight of the 'why', she did a really good job on the whole, and her diligent reporting set us up for what was to become a pivotal moment.

'*So what did you learn about yourself during these past 10 days?*' I asked Marilyn.

'*Hmm... I've learned that I love eating what I want, especially because I don't have to think about it, but I don't always make good choices when I do, and then don't feel so good,*' she replied. '*So I'm still confused!*'

I explained that I could see why she would say that, but that actually she *did* now have some clarity on which to build. Effectively she had now clearly learned that moving forward, no matter what she ate, would mean choosing foods that fulfilled her emotionally, nourished her physically and made sense intellectually. These were the foods that would bring her the peace, poise and clarity that she really needed to be able to make headway in her life.

'*It's the last part that I have trouble with,*' Marilyn reminded me. '*I don't even know what makes sense to me intellectually any more – beyond the basic, "Eat as many fresh fruits and vegetables as you can," of course...*'

'*I know,*' I said, '*which is why that part comes last.*' I continued, '*While it is important that you can believe that what you're eating is good for you, the most important two considerations for a Confused Eater, and especially at this stage, are for you to tune in to your body and emotions, and make sure that those two are completely happy. Then you'll know what foods to eat.*' This made sense to Marilyn, who gladly took it on board for the next week until we spoke again.

One week later and Marilyn had experienced a breakthrough: '*I applied everything we spoke about. But not only that, I started applying the rule not just to what I ate, but to other things in my life. I started making choices that felt good to me and doing other things that I loved and made me feel good; not necessarily ones that I thought I should, or that someone else would tell me to do, and I really got it!*'

While this was just the start of our work together, and Marilyn went on to make great strides in all areas of her life during our time, it was this breakthrough and truly 'getting' the idea that knowledge comes from within, that turned this Confused Eater into a Conscious, Intuitive and, eventually, a really very happy eater!

The Benefits of Being a Confused Eater

Being confused is rarely beneficial! However, there can be *some* plus sides so long as confusion reigns only for a short while.

- Allows you to take time out to reassess your diet and lifestyle.

- If your previous way of eating hasn't been working for you, taking a step back to decide what to do next.

- Eating the way you used to eat once upon a time and re-learning some lessons!

Adopting the Habits of a Confused Eater

- Only choose 'Confused' if you see it as a resting place to reassess or redefine your diet, or even who you are.

- When you're in that place, don't let it bring you down but aim to move out of it quickly with focus and purpose.

- Get clear on what you really want your diet to do for you.

- Set about discovering or creating that diet for yourself.

- Stop listening to everyone else and start listening to yourself.

Integrating with Other Types

Integrated with the Functional Eater

Integrating with the Functional Eater is a good and sensible move for the Confused Eater in that it will enable them to simplify their eating habits, start paying closer attention to what is and isn't working for them as an individual, and (hopefully) find clarity as a result. Because of the level of impact this integration could affect, this is one of the types that could really make all the difference if the Confused Eater is good and ready for change.

Integrated with the Sensual Eater

If the Confused Eater finds the idea of eating for fun and pleasure attractive, then this particular integration could be just the thing to buy them some valuable 'distraction' time. Although this wouldn't usually be considered an evolution for most types, for the Confused Eater, moving out of confusion and into anything that feels tangible and solid and joyful can be seen as an upgrade and help pave the way to even greater evolutions in the future.

Integrated with the Intellectual Eater

Oftentimes what makes for a Confused Eater in the first place is too much intellectualizing, so to integrate *intentionally* with an Intellectual Eater would only be a good idea if what was learned was integrated methodically and without angst. For any Confused Eater to make this integration without having this agreement in place first is likely to lead to even greater confusion, so this is most definitely a case of 'make this choice wisely or don't make it at all.'

Integrated with the Emotional Eater

Mixing the Confused Eater with the Emotional Eater is quite possibly the most unhelpful combination of all. This is because both types are in a place of instability – one intellectually, the other emotionally, and absolutely, in this instance, opposites should not attract. Should this unfortunate pairing happen, the net result can only be stress and upset of epidemic proportions. Simply do not go here.

Integrated with the Focused Eater

This integration is *the* one that could pull the Confused Eater out of intellectual disarray and into focused, passionate action – which is really what they need the most. Perfect for the Confused Eater who is truly serious about moving out of confusion and into clarity, this choice is actually very simple to make, but in doing so asks the Confused Eater to drop the identity they have got so used to, and step into a level of power and responsibility which they may never have experienced before. For the Confused Eater who can do this, a new level of awareness and freedom awaits.

Integrated with the Intuitive Eater

Asking the Confused Eater to get intuitive will result in one of two possible outcomes: they'll either take to it like a duck to water because it gets them out of their head and into their body (and they'll love it), or they'll intellectualize the process too much, decide it's even more complicated than what has gone before, and end up feeling even more confused and overwhelmed than ever. As such, this integration is only recommended if the Confused Eater concerned has the ability simply to 'feel' what's right for them and act on it, as opposed to processing it intellectually or via a filter which might be their latest guru's recommendation.

Integrated with the Conscious Eater

For the Confused Eater who genuinely feels passionate about specific ethical, spiritual, political or environmental concerns, this is a great integration as it will effectively bump a whole lot of options right off their metaphorical plate. One of the issues that Confused Eaters have is that their options are too broad. Having listened to endless debates about what's healthy and what's not, they tend to get to a place where it's all so confusing that anything goes. The path to success, whatever they desire, is to trim down those options to ones that are more personal and more helpful. Integrating with the Conscious Eater can make this happen in a very meaningful and efficient way, with (usually) no questions getting in the way to spoil the process.

Integrated with the Experimental Eater

Imagine taking someone who is already feeling confused and overwhelmed about what – and what not – to eat, and then adding into the mix someone who considers just about any food 'fair game'. This is what you would create with this particular pairing. Could this integration be like putting fuel on the fire, then? Absolutely it could, but it could also create such an extreme experience that the same fire would burn even brighter and even longer to create a phoenix-rising-from-the-ashes type of experience. Imagine letting go of all intellectual ideas and memories about what foods are 'right' and 'wrong' and moving purely into experience. This is a completely viable option, of immense value if the Confused Eater in question is ready for a complete transformation and to leave old ways completely behind.

Integrated with the Social Eater

This is the integration to make when the Confused Eater is ready to 'let it all hang out', try new things (foods and ways of eating) and socialize, both for the pure pleasure of it but also, potentially, to speak to different people about what works for them. As Confused Eaters suffer the most when they stay in their head, any type that enables them to break free of that – and the Social Eater is definitely one of these – is going to give them the opportunity to take a big step back, try something new and potentially open doors to new ways of gaining the all-important joy, peace and clarity.

The Conscious Evolution of the Confused Eater

The Confused Eater is primarily tuned in to their mind, although things can get pretty emotional from time to time.

- **In its weakest expression:** feels continually in a state of confusion and frustration, yo-yo-ing from one fad diet or eating programme to another.

- **In its highest expression:** you use the space of 'confusion' lightly, seeing it as a place you can go to internally when you want to start afresh with your opinions, beliefs and behaviours around food.

The ultimate evolution for the Confused Eater is to shift completely out of confusion and into clarity via embodying the following Eater Types: Sensual + Intellectual + Conscious + Intuitive + Focused.

When the Confused Eater does this they create the experience of:

- loving the food they eat
- knowing that what they are eating is great for them
- feeling genuinely happy with their food choices from an ethical standpoint
- being more tuned in to their body and what *it* wants

- reaching/maintaining their personal health/body goals, whatever these may be.

See pages 253–55 for some great food ideas for the healthy Confused Eater.

SIGNATURE DISH FOR THE CONFUSED EATER

mono melon Smoothie

This recipe is perfect for the Confused Eater because there's only one ingredient, there's no question that it's good for you and you have to drink it on its own because that's the way melon needs to be ingested. Bottom line: it's about as simple as you can get – but, wow! How dreamy it tastes! Simple yet profound.

Serves   1–2

Equipment   Blender

Ingredients 1 ripe melon of your choice (Galia is my favourite melon for this recipe)

Directions

- Simply cut your melon in half and spoon the ripe flesh out of the skin, putting the seeds to one side. If you are serving one person, half a melon will be enough, unless that person is very hungry.

- Blend your melon on high speed until no lumps remain.

KAREN'S TIPS

This is a great breakfast as it is just fruit. If drinking this at any other time of day, to avoid gas and bloating you must drink it on an empty stomach, as all fruits are digested quickly, but melon is the fastest – and when blended faster still! So wait at least three hours after eating your last meal to drink this – hence the breakfast suggestion.

This one won't keep well in the fridge, so best to drink it as soon as possible.

THE SOCIAL EATER 🍎

The Social Eater is a naturally friendly type who loves nothing more than to socialize and have fun around food and drink. Consequently they may be prone to eating whatever it is that's being offered, with far less thought to what it is and why they're eating it than is true of any other type. For the Social Eater the enjoyment of food rests largely on whom it is being enjoyed with, so if company is not available then the TV or radio, or perhaps a book or magazine, may be joining them at the dinner table because it's just not fun eating alone.

For the Social Eater life is one big party, where the order of the day is food, fun, friends and festivity.

The Social Eater's view –

- on food: 'Enjoyable'

- on eating: 'Fun'

- on self-catering: 'Rare'

- on takeaways: 'Conditional'

- on being personally catered for: 'OK'

- on eating out: 'Yippee!'

- on changing their diet: 'As long as I can keep socializing, doing what I do, that could be OK...'

The Social Eater and Pleasure

Social Eaters love it when...

- **they get invited out for dinner or to any social gathering involving food.** Social Eaters are always looking for an excuse to dine out, for myriad reasons. Because they have a wide social circle and because they're highly unlikely ever to say 'No,' you can guess that they'll be dining out anything between one and seven times per week.

- **they come up with a delicious recipe or menu plan which they can serve at their next dinner party.** Social Eaters are not necessarily ones to spend lots of time mixing and blending in the kitchen, because they'd far rather be talking on the phone, reading a book or watching TV – but the one thing that *will* get them excited about pulling out a recipe book will be the thought of creating food with the specific intention of impressing and entertaining others.

- **someone calls round unexpectedly.** There may not be a lot of food in the house, but you can get bet that the Social Eater will find something to rustle up to keep a visitor happy and munching away for an hour or four. For this reason, don't be surprised if you find a secret stash of biscuits hidden in a kitchen cupboard 'just in case'. This will generally be their favourite part of the kitchen and one they keep stocked up with a sense of pride and passion.

The Social Eater's idea of heaven: 'Staying at an all-inclusive retreat, where impressive communal meals are served five times per day and there's evening entertainment.'

The Social Eater and Pain

Social Eaters struggle when…

- **no one wants to come out and play this week.** A day or two they can manage, but if it gets to Wednesday and there's been no breakfast meetings, no lunches with friends, no romantic dinners nor any friends popping round after work, then this is when life starts to feel very awry for the Social Eater.

- **they try to get healthy and it makes a difference to where they can eat.** Heaven forbid that the topic of healthy eating should become a serious consideration for the Social Eater, because this invariably will mean *change*. Just think of all those restaurants that will now be off-limits, or the wine bars that can no longer be frequented. This will be how the Social Eater sees it, at least. The good news is that there is always a way to eat healthily or make better choices than normal, no matter where you are, so this is usually more of a fear-based projection than a real-life scenario.

- **they have to spend a significant amount of time alone.** When this occurs something powerful can happen to the Social Eater. Ordinarily defined by their social life and being in the company of others, time spent alone can result in the Social Eater having the valuable opportunity to get to know themselves better and start to ask bigger questions of *themselves* and their life – so long as they can keep the TV and radio switched off!

The Social Eater's idea of hell: 'Camping solo in a wood with no transport, electricity, people or amenities for miles.'

If This Is You

If you are a Social Eater, or if this fits part of your Eater Type profile, bookmark this page for a second and turn to Chapter 2 (page 126), where there are three short but revealing questions to consider. These questions will help you get more in touch with how being a Social Eater has worked for you *and* caused issues. You don't have to do anything with this information just yet, but don't skip it; it is vital. Take this opportunity to reflect on things; you may well have one or two 'Aha!' moments that could be of tremendous value to you. Once you've done that, come back to this page and keep reading.

. . . .

Case Study: Paul, 39, Los Angeles

Paul's reason for contacting me was simple: he wanted to get 'sharper'. By this he meant that he wanted to up his game both personally and professionally, to get an edge at work and in sport. He was approaching the big 4-0, and was tired of feeling mediocre.

Discovering Paul's personal Eater Type profile was a pivotal moment indeed, as we learned that he was a Social Eater (2) combined with a Sensual Eater (2) and an Experimental Eater (1).

It is not uncommon for someone to comprise two or three types, but when someone's goal is not easily aligned with their current Eater Type profile, that's when things can be a little more tricky.

This was definitely the case with Paul, as none of these types is renowned for being especially focused or edgy! After learning more about the three types that made up his current Eater Type profile, Paul saw clearly that he was going to have to change.

We began by getting really clear and specific about how exactly he wanted his 'edge' to show up. 'How will you know when you've arrived?' I asked. Paul did a great job at getting very clear, very quickly. He plainly wanted what he said he wanted – an excellent sign, as his level of commitment would be the critical factor in how well he transitioned from one Eater Type profile to another.

'That's brilliant,' I said. *'Now on to looking at why you love what you love.'*

We spent some time analysing what exactly it was about each of his three current Eater Types that he loved so much. In Paul's words, this amounted to *'camaraderie'* (Social), *'decadence'* (Sensual) and *'diversity'* (Experimental).

At this point we now had all that we needed to work out a plan. We were looking to build all of the factors that Paul loved into the new, improved eating plan that would get him where he wanted to go.

And so it was that the Focused, Intellectual, Sensual version of Paul was born. By making sure that his social needs were met through sport and eating at healthy eateries with like-minded friends, and creating a menu plan that was interesting, unique and diverse, we were off to a flying start. The final piece of the puzzle was now to find a way that Paul could indulge himself without losing his newly acquired edge, so we kept moving with the theme of looking after his increasingly toned body and he gave himself full permission to get a full body massage at the end of every working week. (Now that's what I call indulgence!)

Three months later and my final call with Paul reflected his level of transformation. Not only had Paul acquired the edge he had wanted so badly for himself, but a smart and beautiful young woman he had had his eye on at the gym had just said 'Yes' to a date with him, and was meeting him for a drink five short hours later.

The Benefits of Being a Social Eater

- Can help you to make new friends.

- Trying new foods and new ways of preparing and presenting meals.

- Learning to combine your lifestyle with your social life.

- Getting out more!

- Opening yourself up to new people and experiences.

Adopting the Habits of a Social Eater

- Mark a diary date to eat out and invite at least two friends.

- Organize an afternoon tea or potluck.

- Book yourself on to a cookery class or other food-related event.

- Make plans for a celebratory birthday or Christmas meal.

- Create an exciting menu plan for a dinner party and then announce it.

Integrating with Other Types

Integrated with the Functional Eater

This wouldn't be the most appealing or obvious integration for the Social Eater to consider, but if they wanted to start taking better care of their body by keeping things simple and easing up on the overindulgence, then integrating with the Functional Eater would absolutely be the way to go. As the Functional Eater is not the biggest fan of eating out, this combination would be very sobering for the Social Eater, both literally and metaphorically. It wouldn't mean the end of social eating, but it would certainly create some food for thought about how often, and the what, when, who and why that lay behind the desire to eat in company so often.

Integrated with the Sensual Eater

If the Social Eater is ready to go gourmet, upscale, decadent and get even *more* excited about food, then this would be the way to go. By combining the Sensual Eater's natural love of all things rich, indulgent and delicious, with the Social Eater's desire to eat out, celebrate and socialize, this is certainly the fast-track to the high life… but it might also be the fast-track to weight gain and focusing on food way more than is healthy for mind or body.

Integrated with the Intellectual Eater

For making healthy choices while still retaining the freedom to party, the combination of Social Eater and Intellectual Eater is a great integration to consider for a healthy balance of food and fun. The Intellectual Eater, having clear opinions on what's 'good' and not-so-good to eat and drink, knows enough to be useful and beneficial to any Eater Type, but is especially good for the Social Eater, because the latter isn't particularly attached to any style of eating so can take on board anything that the Intellectual Eater has to say. A smart move for the party person who wants to wine and dine beyond 50 without health issues.

Integrated with the Emotional Eater

Take a Social Eater and combine them with an Emotional Eater and you create someone who becomes even more dependent on others for emotional support, or someone who starts overeating in public or secretly bingeing in private. In any of these scenarios, there is little joy to be had. Much better to choose a type that's uplifting and has a purpose if they want to stay great company and be able to toast love, life and happiness with sincerity.

Integrated with the Focused Eater

Giving the Social Eater something to aim for is an interesting prospect; after all, socializing is all about being in the moment, and has no specific goal except enjoyment for what is. However, as for any type, integrating with the Focused Eater means that something of meaning gets to be pursued and experienced. If the Social Eater is ready for anything that fits that bill, then this is the integration to go for.

Integrated with the Intuitive Eater

A Social Eater who eats intuitively is a happy one because they feel that they are eating what they want, how they want and when they want. The only curveball is that the Intuitive Eater likes to be more in control of what they eat than the Social Eater, by quite a distance. So, for this to be a union made in heaven, it's important that eateries are chosen with a little bit more sensitivity and consciousness than usual. This way both parts of this integration get to be happy.

Integrated with the Conscious Eater

Integrating with the Conscious Eater is only the right thing to do when the Social Eater is sufficiently moved, and ready, to start making food choices based on 'bigger picture' considerations. Taking into account how often the Social Eater eats out and socializes, this, of course, is no small deal. It needs to be a firm decision and one made with heart and soul if they want to maintain integrity *and* enjoy their mealtimes and dinner conversations for the long haul.

Integrated with the Experimental Eater

When the Social Eater integrates with the Experimental Eater, good times are had. Suddenly things that were off the menu for whatever reason are now very much on the menu, because it's time to try the previously untried and explore the previously unexplored. For the Social Eater who wants to expand their eating experience beyond the norm and open up to new gastronomic adventures, this is the way to go. For the Social Eater who is looking to evolve internally rather than externally, it's fairly safe to say that, as fun as this integration has the potential to be, enlightened eating probably will not be the result.

Integrated with the Confused Eater

Going out to eat and not being able to decide what to eat or why is going to result in the Social Eater becoming the unsociable eater if they're not careful. Part of the Social Eater's charm and joy stems from their carefree and open attitude to food, so bringing the Confused Eater into the mix is never going to add anything of value. Better simply to dabble with the Confused Eater once in a blue moon, when the biggest choice you have to make is between chocolate torte and strawberry shortcake. Don't let it get any bigger or badder than this.

The Conscious Evolution of the Social Eater

The Social Eater is primarily tuned in to their emotions, as they are driven by their pursuit of joy and community.

- **In its weakest expression:** surrenders any level of consciousness around food in favour of being popular, busy and surrounded by others.

- **In its highest expression:** you adore creating and enjoying the best possible food, drink and experiences with those you love, and in doing so bring a great deal of joy to the lives of others.

The ultimate evolution for the Social Eater is to move beyond making food choices based purely on sharing space and time with someone else, to create their future food choices by embodying the following Eater Types: Sensual + Intellectual + Conscious + Intuitive + Focused.

When the Social Eater does this they create the experience of:

- loving the food they eat

- knowing that what they are eating is great for them

- feeling genuinely happy with their food choices from an ethical standpoint

- being more tuned in to their body and what *it* wants

- reaching/maintaining their personal health/body goals, whatever they may be.

See pages 253–55 for some great food ideas for the healthy Social Eater.

SIGNATURE DISH FOR THE SOCIAL EATER

raspberry passion pudding

This recipe is perfect for the Social Eater, because it's a dessert or summer brunch recipe that's universally adored, can be decorated any way you like for the wow factor and, better still, takes only a couple of minutes to make. Well, we wouldn't want to keep you from your guests now, would we?

Serves 1–2

Equipment Blender

Ingredients 3 cups frozen raspberries

1 passion fruit (cut in half and seeds squeezed out, shell discarded)

1 mango, peeled and pitted

Directions

- Place the prepared fresh fruit into the blender first, then add the frozen raspberries on top.

- Blend all ingredients until the mixture is smooth and creamy with no lumps.

- Taste-test before serving. If too tart for your palate, add some honey or dates to your blend.

KAREN'S TIP

Feel free to add any other fresh fruits of your choice and decorate as desired.

CHAPTER 2
So How's That Working For You?

Once you've read about each of the Eater Types, it's time to reflect on the pros and cons of each in relation to the results you've been getting and your 'ultimate 100' result revealed to you via the Ultimate Eater Quiz in Chapter 1.

By the end of this exercise you will be super-clear about what's been working, what's been unhelpful, what specifically needs to be enjoyed and/or evolved more, and what needs to be *eradicated*. Once you know all of this it will become clear how to adopt the habits and thinking of the Eater Type (or combination of Eater Types) that suit/s you best.

Bottom line: this is all about helping you create *the* magic formula that will transform your diet and eating habits into an experience that ticks all the boxes that matter to you, and, *better still*, that you adore.

So, to begin, write down the name/s of the different type/s of eater that you are, in order of dominance. For example if in the What Type of Eater Are YOU? quiz you scored 1 x Functional Eater, 3 x Intellectual Eater and 1 x Intuitive Eater, then Intellectual Eater would be your 'Eater Type #1'. The remaining types, Functional and Intuitive, would then fall in whatever order you decide.

Once you've done that, go ahead and answer the three questions below, taking into account everything you have learned about your type so far, and your own personal experience.

Once you feel you have an answer to the third question about what you need to do, refer back to the section in Chapter 1 for that particular type and read through from the Case Study onwards. This will give you everything you need to be able to address the fourth and final question on page 128 ('Which Eater Type profile would support me best?'), as you'll know what type will best support you in achieving your desired transformation.

It is possible (though rare) that you have chosen a different letter for each of the five questions in the 'What Type of Eater re You?' on pages 9–12, and therefore have five different Eater Types that resonate for you. On the flipside, you might be someone who has only one type – that is, you might have chosen the same letter for all five questions. Whatever your answers may be, just go ahead and answer the following three questions for each of the Eater Types that make up your unique Eater Type profile:

1. **How is this working well for me? Consider this from a physical, emotional, mental, spiritual, financial and practical perspective.**

2. **How is this causing problems for me? Again, think physically, emotionally, mentally, spiritually, financially and practically.**

3. **What do I need to do (specifically) to strengthen the positives and eliminate the negatives?**

Here is an example of how your answers might look if your dominant type is the Sensual Eater:

How Is This Working Well for Me?

Thinking physically, emotionally, mentally, spiritually, financially and practically:

- I love my food!

- I enjoy being 'naughty' with food.

- I like trying new things and experiencing new sensations.

- I like not having any reins on what I eat.

- I am never boring or dull about food because I will try almost anything that tastes good.

How Is This Causing Problems for Me?

Thinking physically, emotionally, mentally, spiritually, financially and practically:

- I do not have the best level of health and vitality.

- I don't feel good in my skin a lot of the time due to my excess weight.

- Because of my weight I can't buy the types of clothes or outfits that I'd really like to wear.

- Sometimes I feel greedy and that my eating can get a little out of control.

- I can sometimes be fussy around food because I like it to be a certain way, and this can annoy friends and family.

What Do I Need to Do?

Thinking about how to strengthen the positives and eliminate the negatives:

- Only eat foods I adore.

- Make a list of my favourite 'naughty' foods and be sure to eat one every day.

- Try at least one new food a week.

- If I create any rules to help me get where I want to go, then they are my rules and not anybody else's.

- Create a menu plan to help me lose the 14 lb I want to lose and get the level of health and energy that I want, while still eating foods I love and 'naughty' foods.

- Take up a new hobby to take my mind off food.

- Give myself a reward for losing the excess weight – like one of those outfits I am desperate to look, and feel, fantastic in.

- List some foods and meals that I would be happy to eat no matter where I am in the world so I do not fuss and irritate others around food.

Now go back to the Case Study (in Chapter 1) for your dominant Eater Type, and read the rest of the chapter from there.

The final question to consider, once you have been through all of Chapter 1, is:

4. Which Eater Type profile would support me best?

In the example of the Sensual Eater, here's what this would look like:

The Eater Type profile that would best support me to experience all I want would be Sensual Eater + Focused Eater.

Here is another example, this time of how your answers might look if your dominant type were Intuitive Eater.

How Is This Working Well for Me?

- I like being spontaneous with food.

- I like not being tied to rules.

- I like letting my body decide what it wants.

- I like being open to new types of awareness without a rule book refraining me from going there.

- I learn a lot of things about myself and where I'm at in my life by allowing my Intuitive Eater to show me what's what.

How Is This Causing Problems for Me?

- Because there are no rules, I am sometimes choosing foods I don't feel consciously or intellectually happy about.

- I have no way of knowing if my intuition is really my intuition, or a craving, or… what?

- I actually used to enjoy having some rules that I followed and could be intuitive about. This created a framework for me so I felt better about myself and I got better results.

What Do I Need to Do?

- Make a complete list of foods that the Intellectual Eater in me knows to be good for me and that the Conscious Eater in me would be happy with.

- Choose a goal for myself that gets me really excited and makes sticking to my framework a necessity as well as a choice.

- Journal daily to connect with myself and what is going on for me.

Which Eater Type Profile Would Support Me Best?

- Intuitive Eater + Focused Eater + Intellectual Eater + Conscious Eater

Once you have completed this exercise, it's time to move things to a much more thought-provoking level…

CHAPTER 3
Everything Changes Right Here

It's All About Energy

As you have learned, knowing what is working for you and what isn't is vital. This is the first step on the path to experiencing the level of food freedom that you really desire.

Congratulations! You've taken care of that part. Already you should be feeling so much clearer and more in touch with yourself.

You are officially halfway through this life-changing process.

What we come to now is something that's set to change the way that you see food and eating forever; lessons that it has taken me nearly two decades of committed study and observation to truly realize and learn.

It's time to talk about *energy*.

I want you to imagine yourself right now as a ball of pure, untainted energy. Forget what your parents named you, or where you live, or the car that you drive or the job that you do – in fact, just let go of everything that you think you are, or anything that takes you away from the truth that underneath all of that, you are…

A bundle of pure, unlimited life-force energy.

Welcome home!

Now, please bear with me for a moment here…

Next, I want you to think of a piece of food. Any food will do. Have it be the first item of food that comes to mind, and hold it firmly in your thoughts.

Here, too, in this food you have a bundle of energy, because everything that exists in this universe is energy, right? *Just like you.*

The thing that I want you to understand the most here, is that if you take one bundle of energy (you) and add into it another bundle of energy (food, drink or any other substance), something gets to happen.

Whatever substance you choose, even if it's just plain water, something is going to happen, period.

And this substance might affect you positively, or negatively – or both, because any substance we put into our body interacts with our energy on many levels.

It changes our physiology and the quality and health of our cells. It affects our emotions – it can take us up, make us go a little crazy, level us out or bring us down. It affects the clarity and quality of our thoughts, and as a result of that, the decisions that we make, the things that we do and the life we effectively create for ourselves. It also affects our level of connection to the self, others, the planet and spirit. And ultimately, it joins *with you* to become part of this bundle of energy called YOU.

Pretty powerful stuff, I'm sure you'll agree.

The fact of the matter is, whatever you put into your body *does* become you – and it affects you way more than any of us could ever possibly know. Just one piece of bread, chocolate, cheese or potato sends a ripple effect throughout your entire being and sets the scene for just about everything that happens next in your life.

Yes, it's *that* BIG!

Now, you may be wondering what this really means for you. After all, this is not the way that food and diet are taught to us in school (if we are taught about them at all), is it?

We get told that we need to eat this or that, or not eat this or that and, if we're lucky, we get to learn about calories, nutrients and how to create a 'well-balanced' diet. And that's where our food education generally ends.

And while all of this is useful to a certain extent, it certainly is not even *half* of the picture.

The truth is that, as energetic beings living in an energetic world, everything that we bring into us – whether it's a substance like a food or drink, or a thought, or a feeling, or something that we read or see on TV – all of this changes our energy at a fundamental level, and from that moment forward, so many other things automatically change, too.

Meet Nancy. Nancy wants to lose weight. She knows that chocolate is a weakness and she has a tendency to overeat cheese. She also knows that when she eats more salads and snacks on veggies rather than bread, she loses weight pretty quickly. Nothing especially new here, right?

But let's go a little deeper.

Let's watch Nancy go to the fridge now and reach for today's first piece of cheese, and listen in on what she and the other aspects of herself have to say about it...

'Mmmm, cheese! I know I shouldn't but this one little piece won't hurt, will it?'

Nancy's body: 'Oh yes it will! I do NOT do well on cheese – and you know it. Except you won't admit it, even though I cough up mucous, break out in spots and end up holding yet more excess fat – that you say you want to get rid of!'

Nancy's emotion: 'And I'm not thrilled about it either. Because every time you eat it I end up getting upset. First because it upsets Body, which always upsets me, and second because I'm going to be all over the place and feeling low after you've eaten it – as usual.'

Nancy's head: 'Right on, Emotion. *I* know it's not that great for any of us as well. You only have to read a decent health or diet book to know that – although there's a few nutrients in there that she could probably do with – but she's been bitten by the desire bug and I'm not sure what any of us can do to stop her…'

Nancy's soul: 'Oh, why do you do it to yourself, Nancy? With every part of you clearly telling you that this isn't a perfect food for you, why would you still consume it? And how are you ever going to hear my great ideas for how you can let go of it and get that body that you really want, if you won't sit still long enough to hear anything that any of us ever has to say?'

What Happens Next…

Even though every part of Nancy (apart from her unconscious self) knows that eating cheese isn't going to benefit her, she still goes ahead and does it.

Sound familiar?

And as soon as she does so, here's what happens next:

Nancy: 'Ugh. Why did I do that? I feel really bad now.'

Nancy's body: 'Surprise, surprise! You have never felt good on cheese, so why on Earth would you do a 180 today? Now I'm feeling tired, grumpy and sick. Thank you so very much – *not*.'

Nancy's emotion: 'I hear you, Body. I am going down, too. And I was just starting to feel positive about helping her lose that weight as well, before the fridge got in the way.'

Nancy's head: 'What *is* up with this? This happens every single time. Now I can't even think clearly enough to bring any kind of inspiration or illumination into her world. It's all I can do to stay any kind of positive at this moment.'

Nancy's soul: 'Sorry, but I've just checked out. If she won't connect with me then obviously I can't connect with her. Everyone knows I don't do shouting. I wish she would just get quiet once in a while to be able to hear my guidance, as I can see much better things for her and what's possible for her, than she can even start to see. You won't believe how much her life could/would be different if she actually tried to access me for once. Maybe one day something will happen to make her actively seek me out...'

As you can see, this is a story that plays out over and over and over again, in people all over the world, every day. Perhaps this has been your story.

There is nothing new here, except to realize that every food or drink choice brings with it a consequence. And when these choices add up over the course of a day, that day could end up looking and feeling abysmal. Or, if all the stars align, physiologically speaking, it could also become a stunning masterpiece.

The Power of Choice

Ask any high achiever what they eat and how they nourish themselves and you will find, without exception, that the quality of food going in is way above our society's norm. It's no coincidence, because they *know* that they too are a product of what they choose to bring into their own personal energy. And because their life means something to them they tend to choose very wisely. For them, the price of making a bad food or lifestyle choice is something they simply don't wish to pay.

So where do we go from here?

First, let's briefly revisit the Eater Types, because now that we can talk about them as they truly are – in energy terms – you'll start to see even more that:

- You do have a choice
- That choice matters

You see, without understanding that the energy you bring into your world has the power to make or break your experience, you could be at risk of seeing your Eater Type/s as something that exist purely and exclusively in your head as simply an idea or concept.

However, actually every Eater Type has its own energy, and each type makes different choices for different reasons. Indeed, every Eater Type has the power to shape your reality in myriad different ways, so you, too, need to choose wisely. Because, for example, when you bring in the energy of the Functional Eater you get to eat purely for hunger and have a very straightforward relationship with food, but when you bring in the energy of the Emotional Eater, you might get to eat anything and everything and create a maelstrom of internal chaos for yourself that you'd really rather do without.

So, just as I want you to be mindful about what foods you bring into your body, for all of the reasons discussed, I also want you to be just as aware that the personality of the Eater Type/s that you bring into your world has just as much power to make or break the experience that you are trying to create for yourself.

In summary:

Who you are being (Eater Type) + What you consume = Your experience

It really is that simple.

To date, if you are like most people, you may have:

- not known who you are being in relation to food

- not been conscious of what you've put into your body or the far-reaching effects of those choices

- not necessarily had any desired outcome for yourself in body and lifestyle terms – or at least, not one that you have 100 per cent committed to and actively pursued with a passion or in complete alignment.

If you have, then you are a very rare person indeed, and you will know that the equation that I've shared with you is the magic formula for getting you where you want to be – because you will have lived it.

Either way, where most people trip up is when, even if they have a goal and know what or what not to eat to get there, they are still missing one very important puzzle piece – and that's to do with identity. Because *who you are being* is absolutely critical to your success – without that part being aligned, then, just like Nancy, every day you run the risk of the slumbering part of you walking into the kitchen or reaching into the cookie jar and mindlessly undoing everything you so dearly want to create.

But that's not going to happen to you anymore, because you have everything you need now to create *exactly* what you want.

So now all you have to do is decide exactly what that is.

It's time to introduce you to The 10 Possibilities.

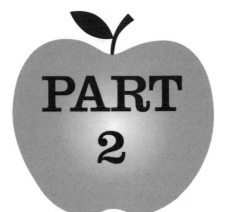

PART
2

the 10
possibilities

CHAPTER 4
The Plate of Possibilities

Knowing your Eater Type profile is one thing, but knowing what to do with it or how to change it (if it's no longer serving you) is another.

This is where all of that starts to change.

So far during our time together you have:

- got clear on what your current relationship with food and eating is like, and how happy you are (or are not) with it

- discovered what your biggest problem is that prevents you from experiencing optimum joy around food and eating

- discovered your score out of the possible 100 in the Ultimate Eater Quiz

- uncovered any themes or patterns around your strengths and weaknesses regarding food

- discovered what your current eater profile is via the What Type of Eater Are YOU? quiz

- learned about each of the different Eater Types, especially your own

- mapped out your own personal Eater Types profile and got super-clear on what's been working within each type, what's been unhelpful, what specifically needs to be enjoyed more, what needs to be eradicated, and what Eater Type (or Types) can best help you to experience that

- learned about food as energy and how that interacts with your own energy to create a new and different experience for you on every level

- learned that you have the power to choose consciously what it is that you want, and that you get to have what you want by first carefully choosing what Eater Type/s you are going to work with and then choosing the foods that you put into your body to get your desired outcome

- started completing your own unique 'Eat Right For Your Personality Type Personal Success Blueprint' – turn to page 257 and complete the first three questions if you haven't done so already.

All of the information you have accrued so far will be invaluable to you as you decide what it is that you really want in this next phase of your life, and how your unique blueprint is going to look to get you there.

By this point, most of the work has been done. Now it's all about choosing.

So what I want you to do now is:

1. get hold of your Blueprint as it exists so far

2. re-read the work you did on page 126 in Chapter 2.

3. answer the following questions so that you can start to create the *energetic* blueprint for what you want to bring into your life.

So with your pen at the ready…

The What Do I Want? Quiz

1. From everything you have learned about yourself so far, what is it that you've been struggling with the most (in relation to food and/or eating) that you are committed to overcoming?

2. From everything you have learned about yourself so far, what is it that you yearn for the most regarding your body/diet/life (that you don't currently have) in order to feel truly happy?

3. From everything you have learned about yourself so far, what is it that you most love about what your current Eater Type/s give you/bring to your life/enable you to experience?

4. From everything you have learned about yourself so far, what is it that you find most frustrating/annoying/debilitating about what your current Eater Type/s give you/bring to your life/lead you to experience?

5. From everything you have learned about the Eater Types and what you want to experience, what new and/or existing Eater Type/s do you think you need to embody to get where you want to be?

6. Taking all of the above into account, which of the following sentences best sums up where you want to go next with your food and eating journey? *Note: choose the one that is the best fit for what you want to experience next. Remember, you can always choose something else in the future, but be where you really are in your life right now and choose what you really want for today and the foreseeable future.*

• I want to discover and embody my perfect size and weight.

• I want to look and feel better.

- I want more energy.

- I want to excel at my chosen sport or personal/professional pursuit.

- I want to experiment and get playful with new foods and ingredients.

- I want to feel at peace.

- I want to eat the healthiest diet possible.

- I want to learn even more about myself.

- I want to nurture and comfort myself right now.

- I want to find a better dietary fit for my current circumstances and lifestyle.

When you have selected your favourite, most desired option from the list above, it's time to introduce you to The 10 Possibilities.

The 10 Possibilities

Here follow The 10 Possibilities of what you can consciously choose to experience about food and eating – specifically, the outcome/reality you want to create for yourself.

1. Eating for Weight Management (Loss or Gain)

2. Eating for Beauty, Health and Vitality

3. Eating for Energy

4. Eating for Performance

5. Eating for Fun and Enjoyment

6. Eating for Peace, Connection and Contentment

7. Eating for Optimum Nutrition

8. Eating for Self-knowledge

9. Eating for Comfort

10. Eating for Convenience, Lifestyle and Circumstance

By this stage you should be in a position to choose the one that feels the most right for where you are at in your life right now. If you don't feel you can do this, ask a friend or loved one to help you go through your answers; it will probably be clear to them what it is that you really want, and they can reflect that back to you.

If you find yourself unable to choose just one Possibility at this stage, that's OK, but you'll want to read through each Possibility in full before finally committing, to see if this remains the case. If it does, don't worry, that's absolutely fine. You should easily be able to find a way to marry two or more different Possibilities together by choosing the best Eater Types to help you get there – but I recommend that pursuing three different Possibilities should be the *absolute maximum*, as it is much easier to focus on creating one reality first and then moving on to a different one later.

So, are you ready to find out more about each different Possibility? Learning more about each one will hopefully bring the clarity that you seek to make a final decision about what you are choosing for yourself, and why.

Enjoy!

EATING FOR WEIGHT MANAGEMENT

Few and far between are those who are entirely happy with their body weight, shape or size. Whether we're carrying too much or too little weight, it can have a significant impact – not just on our physical appearance, but also our emotional and mental well-being and the way we feel about ourselves. Many lives have been blighted by body issues, and continue to be. It doesn't have to be this way.

If you've reached a place where your weight is causing you emotional upset and/or health issues, here would be the perfect place for you to start. When you reach the perfect weight for you, or even get close to it, every area of your life will improve dramatically as you step out of your front door looking good and feeling great with a body that you're finally proud and happy to call home.

Working with your Eater Type could very well be that missing key you've been looking for. Losing or gaining the extra weight will be so much easier when you work in harmony with your natural tendencies and desires, rather than trying to follow someone else's cookie-cutter approach. As you read the action steps for your type, chances are you'll realize where things haven't worked well for you before, and finally you will have a recipe for success on your own terms in your unique, and ultimately winning, style.

Eating for weight management is for you if:

- You want to lose or gain weight to look better
- You want to lose or gain weight to feel better
- You want to lose or gain weight for health reasons
- You want to lose or gain weight for fertility or pregnancy-related reasons
- You want to discover your hottest body ever.

The Eater Types you could run with or integrate for easier weight management:

- **The Functional Eater** – known for eating only when hungry and rarely overeating, so a great ally for staying on the straight and narrow

- **The Sensual Eater** – typically known to indulge, but when used in conjunction with a more grounded and intellectually-inclined type, can give you permission to have those all-important treats and indulgences without going overboard

- **The Intellectual Eater** – can easily find a constructive argument for weight management that becomes a positive force for change

- **The Focused Eater** – excellent at creating a goal and reaching it through planning, commitment and determination

- **The Intuitive Eater** – great at eating only when hungry and having only what the body is really asking for; this lessens the chances of eating foods that aren't supportive of your goals

- **The Conscious Eater** – uses self-control and a powerful personal philosophy to effectively shape eating habits.

Using Your Dominant Type in a Way That Works

Get Clear

Get clear on your goal and write it down – make it a SMART goal, that is: Specific, Measurable, Achievable, Realistic and Timely. Also, imagine how you will look and feel when you get there, and state it in the present tense as if it has already happened:

It is now 31st October 2012 and I weigh 120 lb. I have lost 25 lb in six months and I look and feel amazing. Working with my Eater Type has made it so easy and enjoyable for me. I finally feel as if I have found 'my way' of eating and I love the menus I've created that work with who I naturally am, as well as my lifestyle. I have ditched the diet books for good, discovered what works for me and I truly couldn't be happier!

Put It Up

Put your SMART goal somewhere you can see it every day, multiple times per day. Consider making more than one copy so that you can carry one in your wallet or purse.

Visualize It

See your body the way you really want it. Feel how it feels to have that body. Own it from the inside out. It's already yours… you just have to let go of what you don't need, or add on what you do, depending on whether you need to lose or gain weight.

Commit to It

Commit to doing whatever needs to be done – in a way that works for you. When you follow a plan that works, you will inevitably get the results you desire. Keep reading for how to do just that.

Action Steps

What follows are three powerful action steps for each Eater Type which will help you to reach your target weight specifically in a way that works for you.

If your current eating style is a combination of more than one Type, simply read the action steps for each Type and decide which are going to work best for you. If you'd like to integrate action steps from other Types in order to try out a new Eater Type profile to reach your weight-specific goal, that's absolutely fine. However, do be clear that your main consideration is to be completely honest about what you *know* will work for you, taking into account what you know about yourself, what resonates for you when you read about each Type, and what has occurred in your weight loss/gain story throughout your life so far.

Get a pen and paper to finalize your unique list of action steps. There is a Menu Plan template at the back of this book, or you can also download it for free (together with a special action steps sheet) at ERFYPTBonuses.com, to make the process super-easy and fun.

The Functional Eater

You need a weight-management system that is quick and easy to follow and that involves minimum fuss, tastes delicious and helps you to reach your weight-specific goal simply and easily.

Your Three Best-fit Action Steps

1. List all the foods you want to eat and where to get them (ideally pre-made) so as to make this really easy for you. Next, list the mail order companies, local takeaway places and other super-easy-to-use services that will give you exactly what you want with minimal input on your part.

2. Create or find a menu plan that is quick, easy and delicious to follow, which incorporates these pre-made foods and drinks wherever possible, and includes other meals that you can quickly pull together yourself (in 10 minutes or less) that will help your reach your weight goal.

3. Make three copies of your plan: one for your kitchen, one for your bedroom, one for your wallet or purse. And make sure you stick to it.

The Sensual Eater

You need a weight-management system that satisfies all your senses, is just as pleasurable as your usual menu to eat (or more so) and that enables you to reach your weight-specific goal deliciously and decadently.

Your Three Best-fit Action Steps

1. Buy some new chinaware, glassware or anything for your kitchen that delights and inspires you to symbolize your commitment to a better way and to mark the start of this new phase of your life.

2. Create or find a menu plan that excites you, where everything on your menu feels like a 10/10 for you, including foods and drinks that you consider treats or long-time favourites (these may need to be in a low-fat form or healthier than you are used to, but they can still be just as delicious).

3. Find sensual ways to reward and indulge yourself that are non-edible as you reach your weight-management goals along the way to your final destination.

The Intellectual Eater

You need a weight management system that makes complete sense to you, with no questions left unanswered and that 'adds up' in your head to help you matter-of-factly reach your weight-specific goal.

Your Three Best-fit Action Steps

1. List 10 compelling reasons that *really speak to you* about why you want to or should lose or gain weight.

2. Create or find a menu plan that adds up in a way that makes sense to you, be it calorie-specific, nutritionally sound or whatever criteria naturally speak to you.

3. Set weight loss/gain goals that feel realistic and achievable according to weekly time-frames; create a chart where you can keep track of your progress.

The Emotional Eater

You need a weight-management system that allows you to continue to use food in a way that nurtures you but also makes use of foods that enable you to reach your weight-specific goal comfortably.

Your Three Best-fit Action Steps

1. If you are looking to lose weight: list 10 different non-edible treats that you know will 'fill you up' emotionally. Whenever you find yourself wanting to eat when not hungry, pick one of these treats and enjoy as much as is good for you instead of visiting the fridge or larder.

2. Create or find a menu plan that you feel will keep you happy and full, one that incorporates healthy versions of the comfort foods you are used to reaching for.

3. Ask someone to support you in your weight loss/gain journey by checking in with them daily until you feel you don't need this kind of support anymore. If this isn't something that works for you, spend 15 minutes daily writing in a journal processing your feelings about your day and your eating progress.

The Focused Eater

You need a weight-management system that is to-the-point, easy to follow, that is clearly going to work and enables you to reach your weight-specific goal efficiently and enjoyably.

Your Three Best-fit Action Steps

1. Create a weight-tracker and body measurements chart that clearly maps out your ultimate weight goal, as well as incremental goals, so you can check against them daily/ weekly as appropriate.

2. Create or find a menu plan that you feel confident will get you the results you seek.

3. Invest in whatever tools, support or equipment you need to help you reach your weight goal successfully.

The Intuitive Eater

You need a weight-management system that feels a great fit for you, allows you some flexibility depending on your hunger levels, and enables you to reach your weight-specific goal sensitively.

Your Three Best-fit Action Steps

1. Make a list of foods that your body is asking for right now, and ones that you know your body thrives on the most.

2. Create or find a menu plan comprised of these foods that will also lead to your goals being met.

3. Pay especially close attention to your appetite and physical reactions to foods as you follow your menu plan; tweak it accordingly until you reach your weight-specific goal.

The Conscious Eater

You need a weight-management system that satisfies your soul, is a perfect fit for your highest philosophy and enables you to reach your weight-specific goal easily and peacefully.

Your Three Best-fit Action Steps

1. Make a list of all the foods you are NOT going to eat for the foreseeable future, according to your highest personal philosophy. Then list all the foods that you will feel really good about eating and that you know will support the realization of your goal.

2. Create or find a menu plan that takes these criteria into account, that is created with your weight goal in mind and that makes you feel good on every level.

3. Invest in whatever tools, support or equipment you need to help you reach your weight loss/gain goal successfully.

The Experimental Eater

You need a weight-management system that is as varied as you love things to be, introduces you to new and exciting foods, and allows you to reach your weight-specific goal creatively and enthusiastically.

Your Three Best-fit Action Steps

1. Make a list of all the foods you'd love to try but haven't yet which you know will help you reach your target weight.

2. Create or find a menu plan that incorporates these foods in abundance, as well as your regular favourites (or low-fat versions of them if aiming for weight loss). Make sure your final menu plan feels really exciting to you.

3. Determine how and where you're going to get these foods, and create a plan that enables this to happen easily and joyfully.

The Confused Eater

You need a weight-management system that makes total sense to you, raises no questions whatsoever and that enables you to reach your weight-specific goal confidently and purposefully.

Your Three Best-fit Action Steps

1. Write a list of all the foods and drinks you absolutely KNOW are going to help you reach your weight goal and that you enjoy.

2. Create or find a menu plan that contains these foods – hire a nutritionist or professional healthcare provider to make the plan for you if you feel it's important.

3. Make a commitment with yourself to follow this plan for *at least* two weeks – you can reformat your menu plan after that if you feel you want or need to.

The Social Eater

You need a weight-management system that is fun and flexible to follow, that allows you to socialize as much as you've always done, and that enables you to reach your weight-specific goal joyfully and playfully.

Your Three Best-fit Action Steps

1. Make a list of all the places or social gatherings you love to eat at, are soon to eat at, and want to eat at.

2. Create a menu plan that incorporates these places, the meals you will eat while there, as well as the everyday-at-home foods you like to eat. The two criteria that need to be true for you are that these foods will enable you to reach your weight-specific goal enjoyably while not negatively affecting your social life.

3. Design and host a special dinner party or other food-centred event (a weight-loss/gain group would be great!) that supports your goal in every way, that celebrates your progress to date and that makes you the star of the show. Let your imagination run riot!

Now you've read about each type and the recommended action steps, it's time to write your unique list of action steps which you *know* will get you to your goal in a way that feels great to you.

My Unique Weight-management Plan

Write down your weight loss/gain affirmation. Keep it with you and/or put it up somewhere you can see it every day. Example affirmation: 'I release all excess weight from my body easily, joyfully and completely. I love my new body and I look and feel fantastic!'

Write down your specific 'I am going to love this' action steps.

Now you have your plan, it's time to put it into action.

You can do this! This is your own personal recipe for success – enjoy every second!

EATING FOR BEAUTY, HEALTH AND VITALITY 🍎

Rare is the person who doesn't want to look and feel better – especially as the years march on and wrinkles, lines and grey hairs start to transform a youthful-looking face into a more 'experienced' one! It's not vain or selfish to want to look or feel better. It's a natural inclination. On a deeper level we all know that when our face starts to show age and our health starts to decline, it's a reflection of what's going on inside – a mirror of the corresponding decline in the quality of our blood, tissues and organs.

If the idea of looking and feeling younger is attractive to you, then you're in good company and it's a very wise goal to have. And it isn't actually as hard for you to achieve as you might think. For sure there are foods that are going to enable and disable this Possibility for you (we'll talk more about these shortly), but also, working with your Eater Type can help you enjoy and speed up the process of rejuvenating much more than you can possibly imagine.

Are you ready to play?

Eating for beauty, health and vitality is for you if:

- You want to look better
- You want to feel desirable
- You want to get rid of a niggling health issue
- You want to feel great, consistently
- You want to bounce out of bed in the morning
- You want to bounce back into bed at night.

The Eater Types you could run with or integrate for easier attainment of beauty, health and vitality:

- **The Sensual Eater** – will love working with you from the inside out to help you find the most luxurious, decadent and pampering ways to get your beauty and mojo back.

- **The Intellectual Eater** – can easily find a constructive argument for beauty, health and vitality that becomes its force for change.

- **The Focused Eater** – excellent at creating a goal and reaching it through planning, commitment and determination.

- **The Intuitive Eater** – great for knowing what foods will be the best for leading you to your goal; this lessens the chances of eating foods that aren't supportive.

- **The Conscious Eater** – uses self-control and a powerful personal philosophy to shape eating habits effectively. This will be invaluable in a multitude of ways.

Using Your Dominant Type in a Way That Works

Get Clear

Get clear on your goal and write it down – make it a SMART goal, that is: Specific, Measurable, Achievable, Realistic and Timely. Also, imagine how you will look and feel when you get there, and state it in the present tense as if it's already happened:

It is now 31st October 2012 and when I look in the mirror I love what I see. My daily headaches have gone and when my alarm goes off at 7 a.m. I feel ready to go and no longer have to hit the snooze button. Working with my Type has made it so easy and enjoyable for me. I love the unique approach to looking after myself that I have been able to come up with. It suits me to perfection, both the me that I truly am and the new improved me that I am continually becoming. I am ecstatic!

Put It Up

Put your SMART goal somewhere you can see it every day, multiple times per day. Consider making more than one copy so that you can carry one in your wallet or purse.

Visualize It

See yourself – inside and out – the way you really want to be. Feel how it feels to look in the mirror and love what you see, to feel truly healthy and vital in every cell of your body. Own it from the inside out. It's already yours… you just have to let go of all that isn't serving you and allow your natural birthright of inner beauty and radiance to shine through.

Commit to It

Commit to doing whatever needs to be done – in a way that works for you. When you follow a plan that works, you will inevitably get the results you desire. Keep reading for how to do just that.

Action Steps

What follows are three powerful action steps per Eater Type that will help you to become more beautiful, healthy and vital specifically in a way that works for you. If your current eating style is a combination of more than one Type, simply read the action steps for each Type and decide which action steps are going to work best for you. If you'd like to integrate action steps from other Types in order to try on a new Eater Type profile to reach your specific health and beauty goals, that's absolutely fine. However, do be clear that your main consideration is to be completely honest about what you *know* will work for you, taking into account what you know about yourself, what resonates for you when you read about each Type, and what has occurred in your health and beauty story so far.

Get a pen and paper to finalize your unique list of action steps. There is a Menu Plan template at the back of this book, or you can also download it for free (together with a special action steps sheet) at ERFYPTBonuses.com, to make the process super-easy and fun.

The Functional Eater

You need a beauty, health and vitality plan that is quick and easy to follow and that involves minimum fuss, tastes delicious and helps you to reach your beauty, health and vitality goals simply and easily.

Your Three Best-fit Action Steps

1. List all the fresh fruits, vegetables and other raw foods that you love the most.

2. Create or find a menu plan that is quick, easy and delicious to follow, that incorporates as many of these fresh fruits and vegetables as possible, and includes other high-vitality (ideally 50 per cent+ raw) meals that you can quickly pull together yourself (in 10 minutes or less) that will help you reach your beauty, health and vitality goals.

3. Make three copies of your plan: one for your kitchen, one for your bedroom, one for your wallet or purse. Make sure you stick to it.

The Sensual Eater

You need a beauty, health and vitality plan that satisfies all your senses, is just as pleasurable as your usual menu to eat (or more) and that enables you to reach your beauty, health and vitality goals deliciously and decadently.

Your Three Best-fit Action Steps

1. Find a picture of a person who embodies your desires for beauty, health and vitality, and imagine yourself becoming that person. Use the power of your heart and mind to merge energetically with that vision, so you can connect to it and start to embrace that reality for yourself.

2. Create or find a high-nutrient, high-raw menu plan that excites you, where everything on your menu feels like a 10/10 for you.

3. List 14 different *non-edible* ways that you can indulge your sensuality *and* support your beauty, health and vitality goals. Enjoy one or two of them every day so you feel fully supported and nurtured – or naughty!

The Intellectual Eater

You need a beauty, health and vitality plan that makes complete sense to you, with no questions left unanswered and that 'adds up' in your head to help you reach your beauty, health and vitality goals matter-of-factly.

Your Three Best-fit Action Steps

1. List 10 compelling reasons why becoming more beautiful, healthy and vital are important to you.

2. Create or find a menu plan that is proven to deliver the beauty, health and vitality benefits that you desire.

3. Keep track of your progress on a daily or weekly basis (whatever is the best fit for your schedule) so you can see how things are changing in your face, body and overall sense of well-being.

The Emotional Eater

You need a beauty, health and vitality plan that allows you to carry on using food in a way that nurtures you while using foods that enable you to reach your beauty, health and vitality goals comfortably.

Your Three Best-fit Action Steps

1. List 10 different non-edible treats that you know will 'fill you up' emotionally and make you feel good about yourself. Whenever you find yourself wanting to eat when you're not hungry, or to have something that you know isn't going to help you reach your goals, pick one of these treats and enjoy as much of it as is good for you instead of visiting the fridge or larder.

2. Create or find a high-raw menu plan that you feel will keep you happy and full. Incorporate your non-edible treats into the plan, so you can enjoy one to three of these every day.

3. Ask someone to support you in your beauty, health and vitality journey by checking in with them daily until you feel you don't need that level of support anymore. If this isn't something that works for you, spend 15 minutes daily writing in a journal processing your feelings about your day and your eating progress.

The Focused Eater

You need a beauty, health and vitality plan that is to-the-point, easy to follow, that is clearly going to work and enables you to reach your beauty, health and vitality goals efficiently and enjoyably.

Your Three Best-fit Action Steps

1. Take photos, write detailed notes and record any other important information about your 'before' situation, so that you can capture it accurately and fully. Get really clear on what specific beauty, health and vitality results you are looking to achieve, then put in place a progress chart so you can record and monitor your progress on a daily basis.

2. Create or find a menu plan that you feel confident will get you the results you seek.

3. Invest in whatever tools, support or equipment you need to help you reach your beauty, health and vitality goals successfully.

The Intuitive Eater

You need a beauty, health and vitality plan that feels a great fit for you, allows you some flexibility depending on your hunger levels, and enables you to reach your beauty, health and vitality goals sensitively.

Your Three Best-fit Action Steps

1. Make a list of all the raw fruits and vegetables and other low-fat, raw foods that you know your body thrives on the most.

2. Create or find a menu plan that comprises these foods to a level of 80–90 per cent and that will lead to your goals being met.

3. Pay close attention to how your face, body and overall sense of well-being change as you follow your menu plan, and tweak accordingly until you reach your beauty, health and vitality goals.

The Conscious Eater

You need a beauty, health and vitality plan that satisfies your soul, is a perfect fit for your highest philosophy and enables you to reach your beauty, health and vitality goals easily and peacefully.

Your Three Best-fit Action Steps

1. Make a list of all the raw foods that you know you enjoy and that fit in with your highest personal philosophy.

2. Create or find a menu plan that revolves around these foods, that is created with your most alive version of yourself in mind and that uplifts you spiritually.

3. Spend a few minutes every day connecting with the most beautiful, healthy and vital vision of yourself you can imagine. Bring that vision into every cell of your body through the power of intention and enjoy the 'taking on' of that new reality.

The Experimental Eater

You need a beauty, health and vitality plan that is as varied as you love it to be, introduces you to new and exciting foods, and allows you to reach your beauty, health and vitality goals creatively and enthusiastically.

Your Three Best-fit Action Steps

1. Make a list of all the raw foods that pique your interest and you'd love to try (but haven't yet) and that will add a whole new dimension to your diet.

2. Create or find a menu plan that incorporates these specific foods together with other fresh fruits and vegetables that you love, plus additional low-fat, high-vitality foods that you've never tried before. Through this menu plan, see

yourself setting out on a new adventure, inside and out. Make sure your final menu plan feels really exciting to you.

3. Determine how and where you're going to get these foods, and create a plan that enables this to happen easily and joyfully.

The Confused Eater

You need a beauty, health and vitality plan that makes total sense to you, raises no questions whatsoever and that enables you to reach your beauty, health and vitality goals confidently and purposefully.

Your Three Best-fit Action Steps

1. Write a list of all the raw foods and drinks that you already know you love.

2. Create or find a menu plan that revolves around these foods. Hire a nutritionist or professional healthcare provider to make the plan for you if you feel you need help.

3. Make a commitment to yourself to follow this plan for *at least* one month – you can reformat your menu plan after that if you feel you want or need to.

The Social Eater

You need a beauty, health and vitality plan that is fun and flexible to follow, that allows you to socialize as much as you've always done, and that enables you to reach your beauty, health and vitality goals joyfully and playfully.

Your Three Best-fit Action Steps

1. Find out about all the healthiest eateries local to you (especially juice bars and raw food restaurants and

cafes) and commit to eating *only* there for the next four weeks. If this is not possible, then commit to eating only truly healthy foods at whatever social function/s you are attending during this time period.

2. Create a menu plan that incorporates the meals you will eat while at these places, as well as any raw fruits and vegetables and other raw foods/juices that you like to eat and are happy to eat at home, whether alone or in company.

3. Design and host a special dinner party or other food-centred event that is beauty-, healthy- and vitality-focused so that other people can explore and enjoy this way of eating, too.

Now you've read about each type and the recommended action steps, it's time to write down your unique list of action steps that you *know* will get you to your goal/s in a way that feels great to you.

My Unique Beauty, Health and Vitality Plan

Write down your beauty, health and vitality affirmation. Keep it with you and/or put it up somewhere you can see it every day. Example affirmation: 'With every mouthful I consume I am creating an ever-increasingly radiant face, body and being that wows and delights me.'

Write down your specific 'I am going to love this' action steps.

Now you have your plan, it's time to put it into action.

You can do this! This is your own personal recipe for success – you're going to love watching and feeling yourself becoming rejuvenated from the inside out!

EATING FOR ENERGY 🍎

It's no secret that 80 per cent+ of the Western population complain of 'lack of energy'. Specifically we're talking about having enough energy to get them through their day – that's before wanting energy to do other, more exciting and evolutionary things.

The fact is, our bodies have access to unlimited amounts of energy. We can take it in through the food we eat, the air we breathe, the sunshine absorbed through our skin – even the thoughts that we think or the feelings that we feel can energize us or deplete us, depending on the nature of those thoughts or feelings. It's simply the way that we access it, channel it, manage it and use it that makes the fundamental difference. It could easily be said that learning how to channel energy successfully through our physical body is the number one secret to living a healthy, happy and all-round bountiful life.

If you'd like to experience more energy in your body and consequently your life, then actively and enthusiastically pursuing this particular Possibility will bring you a great deal of invaluable learning, joy and growth. By working with your particular Eater Type or profile you can align with who you are and watch as that expression evolves into something that amazes and excites you beyond measure.

Eating for energy is for you if:

- You feel tired throughout the day

- You're ready for bed at 9 p.m. (or earlier)

- You don't have any spare energy to do other things

- You'd love to be able to exercise or do things at weekends but you'd rather just lay on the sofa and read a book

- You want to get excited about life again.

The Eater Types that you could run with or integrate for gaining more energy:

- **The Functional Eater** – will help you to eat only for hunger and not overindulge, which would rob you of that precious energy you are trying to gain.

- **The Sensual Eater** – will love working with you from the inside out to help you find the most enjoyable and 'naughty' ways to get your energy up and increasing.

- **The Intellectual Eater** – can easily find a constructive argument for gaining more energy that becomes its force for change.

- **The Focused Eater** – will help you create a goal that excites you and help you reach it through planning, commitment and determination.

- **The Intuitive Eater** – will instinctively know what to do and what not to do when you ask for guidance about how best to increase your energy.

Using Your Dominant Type in a Way That Works

Get Clear

Get clear on your goal and write it down – make it a SMART goal, that is: Specific, Measurable, Achievable, Realistic and Timely. Also, imagine how you will look and feel when you get there, and state it in the present tense as if it has already happened:

> *It is now 31st October 2012 and I am thrilled at how much energy I have. I can now stay up until 11 p.m. every night if I want to (sometimes later), I go to the gym three times a week and I am no longer too tired for sex. Working with my Type has made this journey a dream. I love being able to gain more energy through working with who I truly am in this way, and I've*

discovered new aspects to myself along the way. In fact, I love everything about my new life and how I feel in myself, thanks to working consciously on gaining more energy. I am a different, happier, more enthusiastic person and I feel great!

Put It Up

Put your SMART goal somewhere you can see it every day, multiple times per day. Consider making more than one copy so that you can carry one in your wallet or purse.

Visualize It

See yourself – inside and out – the way you really want to be. Feel how it would be to feel energized from your head to your toes and be able to do whatever you want without limitation. Own it from the inside out. Allow yourself to let this Possibility become a reality, because, like everything in life, it is always yours for the taking.

Commit to It

Commit to doing whatever needs to be done – in a way that works for you. When you follow a plan that works, you will inevitably get the results you desire.

Action Steps

What follows are three powerful action steps per Eater Type that will help you to become more energetic and alive specifically in a way that works for you. If your current eating style is a combination of more than one Type, simply read the action steps for each Type and decide which ones are going to work best for you. If you'd like to integrate action steps from other Types in order to try on a new Eater Type profile to reach your specific energy goals, that's absolutely fine. However, do be clear that your main consideration is to be completely honest about what you *know* will work for you, taking into account what you know about yourself, what resonates for you when you read about each Type, and what has occurred in your 'energy history' story so far.

Get a pen and paper to finalize your unique list of action steps. There is a Menu Plan template at the back of this book, or you can also download it for free (together with a special action steps sheet) at ERFYPTBonuses.com, to make the process super-easy and fun.

The Functional Eater

You need an energy plan that is quick and easy to follow and that involves minimum fuss, tastes delicious and helps you to reach your energy goals simply and easily.

Your Three Best-fit Action Steps

1. List all the foods that you love to eat, are quick and easy to prepare (or that you can buy pre-prepared) and that you know are truly good for you and will enhance your energy. Next, list the mail order companies, local takeaways and other super-easy-to-use services that will give you these foods 'good to go' with minimal input on your part.

2. Create or find a menu plan that is quick, easy and delicious to follow, that incorporates these pre-made foods and drinks wherever possible, and includes other meals which you can quickly pull together yourself (in 10 minutes or less) that will help your reach your energy goals.

3. Make three copies of your plan: one for your kitchen, one for your bedroom, one for your wallet or purse. And make sure you stick to it.

The Sensual Eater

You need an energy plan that satisfies all your senses, is just as pleasurable as your usual menu to eat (or more) and that enables you to reach your energy goals deliciously and decadently.

Your Three Best-fit Action Steps

1. List 30 different things you would love to do if you had all the energy you wanted. Make 10 of those fun, 10 decadent and 10 naughty – or list 30 things that are all three of these at once!

2. Create or find a menu plan that is clean, nutrient-dense and that includes enough (but not too many!) high-quality 'naughty' foods to excite you. Everything on your menu needs to feel like a 10/10 for you *and* give you more vitality and energy.

3. Grab your list and reward and indulge yourself with a special energy treat each time you do something that takes you closer to your energy goal, all the way to your final destination.

The Intellectual Eater

You need an energy plan that makes complete sense to you, with no questions left unanswered; one that 'adds up' in your head to help you matter-of-factly reach your energy goals.

Your Three Best-fit Action Steps

1. List 10 compelling reasons, which are really important to you, why you truly want to gain more energy.

2. Create or find a menu plan that adds up in a way that makes it obvious that, with its help, you're going to gain all the energy that you want.

3. Set energy-related goals that feel realistic and achievable according to weekly time-frames, and create a chart where you can keep track of your progress.

The Emotional Eater

You need an energy plan that allows you to continue to use food in a way that nurtures you, but one using foods that enable you to reach your energy goals comfortably.

Your Three Best-fit Action Steps

1. Find 12 different *healthy* 'energy-enhancing' foods that you know will also feel comforting to you.

2. Create or find a menu plan that comprises 80 per cent clean, healthy foods, and 20 per cent comforting foods from the list you made for step 1.

3. Spend 15 minutes daily writing in a journal, processing your feelings about your day and the changes in energy that you are experiencing. Allow whatever is showing up for you to come out.

The Focused Eater

You need an energy plan that is to-the-point, easy to follow, that is clearly going to work and enables you to reach your energy goals efficiently and enjoyably.

Your Three Best-fit Action Steps

1. Create a way of measuring and monitoring your energy, in whatever way works best for you, so you can check against it on a daily basis.

2. Create or find a menu plan that you feel confident will bring you the amount of energy (and type of energy) that you seek.

3. Invest in whatever tools, support or equipment you need to help you reach your energy goals successfully.

The Intuitive Eater

You need an energy plan that feels a great fit for you, enables you some flexibility depending on your hunger levels, and enables you to reach your energy goals sensitively.

Your Three Best-fit Action Steps

1. Make a list of foods that you know your body historically has always thrived on and that increase rather than deplete your energy.

2. Create or find a menu plan that revolves around these foods and will deliver the level and type of energy that you desire.

3. Pay close attention to your energy levels as you follow your menu plan, tweaking meals and ingredients accordingly until you reach your energy goals.

The Conscious Eater

You need an energy plan that satisfies your soul, is a perfect fit for your highest philosophy, and enables you to reach your energy goals easily and peacefully.

Your Three Best-fit Action Steps

1. Make a list of all the foods that you know or intuitively feel will have a positive impact on your energy levels (on every level).

2. Create or find a menu plan that revolves around these foods, that is aligned with your highest energetic vision for yourself and that brings you the quality and quantity of energy that you desire in whatever way you most want it.

3. Spend some quality time with yourself, acknowledging the different types of energy within yourself (physical, mental, emotional and spiritual) and where your energy is at within each of those levels.

The Experimental Eater

You need an energy plan that is as varied as you love it to be, introduces you to new and exciting foods and allows you to reach your energy goals creatively and enthusiastically.

Your Three Best-fit Action Steps

1. Make a list of all the energy-enhancing foods that you've heard of but haven't tried before.

2. Create or find a menu plan that incorporates these foods and gives you plenty of opportunity to experiment. Make sure your final menu plan feels really exciting to you.

3. Determine how and where you're going to get these foods, and create a plan that enables this to happen easily and joyfully.

The Confused Eater

You need an energy plan that makes total sense to you, raises no questions whatsoever and that enables you to reach your energy goals confidently and purposefully.

Your Three Best-fit Action Steps

1. Write a list of all the foods and drinks you absolutely KNOW are going to help you increase your physical energy levels.

2. Create or find a menu plan that revolves around these foods – hire a nutritionist or professional healthcare provider to make the plan for you if you feel it's important.

3. Make a commitment to yourself to follow this plan for *at least* two weeks – you can reformat your menu plan after that if you feel you want or need to.

The Social Eater

You need an energy plan that is fun and flexible to follow, that allows you to socialize as much as you've always done, and that enables you to reach your energy goals joyfully and playfully.

Your Three Best-fit Action Steps

1. Make a list of all the places or social gatherings you know you are scheduled or likely to eat at during the next four weeks.

2. Create a menu plan based on this knowledge, choosing meals that are the most energy-enhancing ones on the menu, and also planning for establishments that can deliver the best quality possible, such as juice and smoothie bars, and super-healthy restaurants, cafes and takeaways.

3. Design and host a special dinner party or other food-centred event with 'energy' as its central theme. This could be an event where the foods are all energy enhancing, there are high-energy games, challenges or dancing, and even where everyone has to arrive on foot, no matter how far away they live.

Now you've read about each type and the recommended action steps, it's time to write your unique list that you *know* will get you to your goal/s in a way that feels great to you.

My Unique Energy Plan

Write your energy affirmation. Keep it with you and/or put it up somewhere you can see it every day. Example affirmation: 'Everything I eat supports increasing amounts of life-force energy to come coursing through my veins!'

Write down your specific 'I am going to love this' action steps.

Now you have your plan, it's time to put it into action.

You can do this! This is your own personal recipe for success – you're going to love having all the energy you desire to live the life you want to live – go for it!

EATING FOR PERFORMANCE

Anyone who is serious about performing brilliantly in whatever they do – athletics, a specific sport, in their career or profession, or even as a lover – knows that what they put into their body has everything to do with what they get out of it. For this reason, if performance is important to you then proactively looking at changing what and how you eat, assuming you approach it in the same way that you approach what you 'perform at', is going to pay off in spades.

This particular Possibility is perfect for those who have already been successful at mastering other aspects of their physical vitality and well-being, such as weight management, energy and health, so if you're looking to up your game and attain mastery at a whole new level, then this particular Possibility will give you lots to think about and plenty of room to explore, refine and grow. By working with your particular Eater Type or profile you can make this entire journey to physical mastery a lot more fun, rewarding and effective than it might otherwise have been.

To perfection!

Eating for performance is for you if:

- You want to excel in a particular area of your life

- You want to be the best you can be

- You know that if you changed your diet your performance would increase dramatically

- You are ready for a new challenge and are excited by it

- You want to see what's possible for yourself.

The Eater Types that you could run with or integrate for improving your performance:

- **The Functional Eater** – great for helping you keep the mindset that food is a source of nutrition rather than something to be indulged in or get emotional about.

- **The Intellectual Eater** – will help you list all the many ways that you and your life will improve as a result of bettering your performance, as well as why that is something well worth pursuing and achieving.

- **The Focused Eater** – will help you create a goal that sees you being where you want to be, and help you reach it through planning, focus, commitment and determination.

- **The Experimental Eater** – will open you up to new ways of doing things to get the best possible results.

Using Your Dominant Type in a Way That Works

Get Clear

Get clear on your goal and write it down – make it a SMART goal, that is: Specific, Measurable, Achievable, Realistic and Timely. Also, imagine how you will look and feel when you get there, and state it in the present tense as if it has already happened:

> It is now 31st October 2012 and my performance on the pitch has never been better. I have been awarded player of the match five times, have been taken out of reserve, and am now seen by the regional newspapers as the man to watch in 2013. Working with my Type has made all the difference. It has meant that I'm no longer fighting against myself to be better, I just am. I never thought I could get where I am, but now I have the secret to doing it, I can see only even greater performance and results for myself in the future. I'm psyched!

Put It Up

Put your SMART goal somewhere you can see it every day, multiple times per day. Consider making more than one copy so that you can carry one in your wallet or purse.

Visualize It

See yourself – inside and out – the way you really want to be. Feel how it would be to be the best at whatever it is you want to be phenomenal at. Own it from the inside out. Allow yourself to let this Possibility become a reality because, like everything in life, it is always yours for the taking.

Commit to It

Commit to doing whatever needs to be done – in a way that works for you. When you follow a plan that works, you will inevitably get the results you desire.

Action Steps

What follows are three powerful action steps per Eater Type that will help you to perform at your best specifically in a way that works for you. If your current eating style is a combination of more than one Type, simply read the action steps for each Type and decide which action steps are going to work best for you. If you'd like to integrate action steps from other Types in order to try on a new Eater Type profile to reach your specific performance goals, that's absolutely fine. However, do be clear that your main consideration is to be completely honest about what you *know* will work for you, taking into account what you know about yourself, what resonates for you when you read about each type, and how you have performed in this area so far.

Get a pen and paper to finalize your unique list of action steps. There is a Menu Plan template at the back of this book, or you can also download it for free (together with a special action steps sheet) at ERFYPTBonuses.com, to make the process super-easy and fun.

The Functional Eater

You need a performance plan that is quick and easy to follow and that involves minimum fuss, tastes delicious and helps you to reach your performance goals simply and easily.

Your Three Best-fit Action Steps

1. List all the foods that you know are likely to help you get clear and support you in reaching your specific performance-related goal. Next, list the foods that you know will prevent you from reaching your goal because of their negative effects on your unique body. Finally, list the mail order companies, local takeaways and other super-easy-to-use services that will give you exactly what you want with minimal input on your part.

2. Create or find a menu plan that is quick, easy and delicious to follow, that incorporates these pre-made foods and drinks wherever possible, and also includes other meals that you can quickly pull together yourself (in 10 minutes or less) that will help you reach your performance goal/s.

3. Make three copies of your plan: one for your kitchen, one for your bedroom, one for your wallet or purse. Make sure you stick to it.

The Sensual Eater

You need a performance plan that satisfies all your senses, is just as pleasurable as your usual menu to eat (or more so) and that enables you to reach your performance goals deliciously and decadently.

Your Three Best-fit Action Steps

1. Decide on what juicy, worth-giving-your-everything-for reward you are going to give yourself when you reach your performance goal.

2. Make a list of all the foods you already love which you know will help you reach your performance goal.

3. Create or find a menu plan that revolves around these foods, with the rest comprising simple, clean, healthy foods that keep your mind and body clear.

The Intellectual Eater

You need a performance plan that makes complete sense to you, with no questions left unanswered; one that 'adds up' in your head to help you matter-of-factly reach your performance goals.

Your Three Best-fit Action Steps

1. List 10 compelling reasons why you want to reach the goal you have set for yourself and all the ways reaching that goal will benefit you.

2. Create or find a menu plan that is specifically geared to improving focus, concentration and stamina.

3. Set performance goals that feel realistic and achievable according to weekly time-frames and create a chart where you can keep track of your progress.

The Emotional Eater

You need a performance plan that allows you to continue to use food in a way that nurtures you but uses foods that enable you to reach your performance goals comfortably.

Your Three Best-fit Action Steps

1. List 10 different non-edible treats that you can use to reward yourself for every milestone you reach on the way to your performance goal.

2. Create or find a menu plan that you feel will support you in the pursuit and attainment of your goal, and that has built-in comfort foods that won't derail your progress.

3. Ask someone to support you in your specific performance journey by talking with or getting coaching from them until you reach your desired destination.

The Focused Eater

You need a performance plan that is to-the-point, easy to follow, that is clearly going to work and enables you to reach your performance goals efficiently and enjoyably.

Your Three Best-fit Action Steps

1. Create a chart that clearly maps out your starting point, your final destination and the in-between, incremental goals you need to reach for attaining your performance-related goal/s. Check against them daily/weekly as appropriate.

2. Create or find a menu plan that you feel confident will get you the results you seek.

3. Invest in whatever tools, support or equipment you need to help you reach your performance goal/s successfully.

The Intuitive Eater

You need a performance plan that feels a great fit for you, enables you to have some flexibility depending on your hunger levels, and enables you to reach your performance goals sensitively.

Your Three Best-fit Action Steps
1. Make a list of foods that you know have always supported you to perform at your best.

2. Create or find a menu plan comprised of these foods and that will also lead to your specific performance-related goal being met.

3. Pay close attention to what foods and drinks sustain your performance, and which ones undermine it. Tweak your eating until you reach your desired goal.

The Conscious Eater

You need a performance plan that satisfies your soul, is a perfect fit for your highest philosophy and enables you to reach your performance goals easily and peacefully.

Your Three Best-fit Action Steps
1. Make a list of all the foods that you feel or know will enhance your performance, ones that you can feel really good and whole about.

2. Create or find a menu plan that revolves predominantly around these foods, with the remaining 20 per cent being what makes you the most happy and/or spiritually connected.

3. Spend time with yourself reflecting and journaling about your personal journey en route to your juicy performance-related goal.

The Experimental Eater

You need a performance plan that is as varied as you love things to be, introduces you to new and exciting foods, and allows you to reach your performance goals creatively and enthusiastically.

Your Three Best-fit Action Steps

1. Make a list of all the foods you'd love to try but haven't yet, and which you know will help you reach your performance goal.

2. Create or find a menu plan that incorporates these foods in abundance as well as your regular favourites. Make sure your final menu plan feels really exciting to you.

3. Determine how and where you're going to get these foods, and create a plan that enables this to happen easily and joyfully.

The Confused Eater

You need a performance plan that makes total sense to you, raises no questions whatsoever and that enables you to reach your performance goals confidently and purposefully.

Your Three Best-fit Action Steps

1. Write a list of all the foods and drinks that you enjoy and that you absolutely KNOW are going to help you reach your performance goal.

2. Create or find a menu plan that contains these foods – hire a nutritionist or professional healthcare provider to make the plan for you if you feel that will help.

3. Make a commitment to follow this plan for *at least* four weeks – you can reformat your menu plan after that if you feel you want or need to.

The Social Eater

You need a performance plan that is fun to follow and flexible, that allows you to socialize as much as you've always done, and that enables you to reach your performance goals joyfully and playfully.

Your Three Best-fit Action Steps

1. Make a list of all the places or social gatherings that will assist you in eating for performance without any stress.

2. Create a menu plan that incorporates these places and the meals you will eat while there, as well as the everyday-at-home foods you like to eat which will also support your performance-related goals.

3. Design and host a special dinner party or other food-centred event that celebrates and embodies the theme of 'performance' and plays into the goal you desire to reach. You can be as basic or outrageous with this as you wish!

Now you've read about each type and the recommended action steps, it's time to write your unique list of action steps that you *know* will get you to your goal/s in a way that feels great to you.

My Unique Performance Plan

Write down your performance affirmation. Keep it with you and/or put it up somewhere you can see it every day. Example affirmation: 'It is easy for me to achieve the level of performance that I want as I stay congruent with what will get me there.'

Write down your specific 'I am going to love this' action steps.

Now you have your plan, it's time to put it into action.

You can do this! This is your own personal recipe for success – you're going to adore being able to perform at the level that you've always dreamed of. Get to it!

EATING FOR FUN AND ENJOYMENT 🍎

Who said that eating has to have a point beyond living in the moment, enjoying every mouthful and eating whatever you want? Probably not any diet or health book you have ever read, but sometimes this is actually a very good place to be.

To be clear, I am definitely *not* saying that eating for fun and enjoyment exclusively is a recipe for a super-healthy life and a model-fit body, because it rarely is! But there are definitely times when it's good to kick back, indulge and 'let it all hang out' for a particular reason, as long as you're clear on exactly why you're doing it.

Times like this usually come during or after periods of unusually high stress, when on holiday, when taking time to reconsider one's life path or position in life. At this point anything goes, until something superior is chosen. For this reason, eating for fun and enjoyment can be just what the doctor ordered, reminding us that sometimes taking off all the labels, ditching all the rule books and doing away with the desire to have more or be more – which can sometimes be so draining – can often be the healthiest thing for your exhausted heart and soul to do.

This particular Possibility is for you if any of the above resonates and you don't want to pursue, push or pressurize yourself right now – you just want to eat what you want to eat and let that be OK. While holistically it's not the best place to stay for more than a short while (because, taken to the extreme you can do your body, and ultimately your whole self, varying degrees of harm), when adopted with a healthy degree of moderation it can be nothing less than perfect.

Eating for fun and enjoyment is for you if:

- You don't want to think about food and what's healthy right now

- You want to explore food without limitations

- You are going through a hard time right now and one more 'to do' on your list will push you over the edge

- You've always eaten according to a rulebook and you want to see what happens when you don't

- You want to know what happens around food and eating when you're left to your own devices.

The types that you could run with or integrate for experiencing more fun and enjoyment with your food:

- **The Sensual Eater** – will give you permission to engage all of your senses and come to enjoy and appreciate food from more than one dimension. This is especially good if historically you've been a Functional Eater.

- **The Intuitive Eater** – will guide you to new foods or ones that keep you healthy while you're experimenting and relaxing with your diet.

- **The Experimental Eater** – will encourage you to try new things, especially things you've never heard of before, 'just to see'.

- **The Social Eater** – will take you to places that you've never been before and introduce you to new eating establishments, people and experiences that could ultimately enrich and improve your quality of life.

Action Steps

There are no action steps for each Eater Type in this Possibility because it literally is as simple as 'Eat what you want, when you want' – but don't forget the advice given at the start of this Possibility!

EATING FOR PEACE, CONNECTION AND CONTENTMENT 🍎

Numerous are those who feel anything *but* peace, connection and contentment around their food and eating experience, and this is very much a malady of the modern age.

The good news is that learning to eat this way is actually so much easier than most people think, but it does usually call for some radical moves. This all stems from the fact that modern food-production methods have taken away a massive piece of the 'connection' part of our eating experience, and with it the peace and contentment aspects as well.

For example, very few people now grow their own food. Most people eat food from a box, tin or packet, and as a consequence very few people take any time whatsoever to connect with their food, think about where it comes from, be grateful for it and eat in a way that feels genuinely loving and respectful.

It goes without saying that creating a respectful, conscious relationship with food is a very beautiful, moving and powerful thing to do. When you learn to eat for peace, connection and contentment, you don't just get to enjoy a higher level of experience and engage more deeply with your food, but the knock-on effects cannot fail to ripple through every other area of your life with similar profundity.

Just imagine what that could really mean for you.

This particular Possibility is for you if you are ready to have a deeper, more meaningful relationship with your food, your body, and yourself. It may not be the easiest path if you are someone who has come to rely on heavily processed and commercialized foods and drinks, but you will certainly never feel more happy or fulfilled by your eating choices than when you make the switch to eating with your heart and soul fully engaged, and get to feel the benefits.

Eating for peace, connection and contentment is for you if:

- You feel anything but peace, connection and contentment with your food choices

- You want to feel integrated and whole

- You are ready to make some radical changes in order to reap massive, far-reaching benefits

- You want to evolve your eating habits so they feel more spiritually aligned

- You are no longer prepared to suffer the things that not eating this way has already cost you.

The Eater Types that you could run with or integrate for experiencing more peace, connection and contentment with your food:

- **The Sensual Eater** – will encourage you to eat foods that are more wholesome, natural and pleasurable so that you don't feel this choice is somehow a lesser one.

- **The Focused Eater** – will support you by creating a vision of the new, more peaceful and connected you that you aspire to be, and give you the guidelines, plan and action steps to get you there.

- **The Intuitive Eater** – will guide you to the foods that will be a great fit for you and your body, and invite you to try new foods that you may have eschewed before.

- **The Conscious Eater** – will work with your heart and soul to create some guidelines that enable you to feel genuinely good about your food choices from a moral, ethical and spiritual standpoint.

Using Your Dominant Type in a Way That Works

Get Clear

Get clear on your goal and write it down – make it a SMART goal, that is: Specific, Measurable, Achievable, Realistic and Timely. Also, imagine how you will look and feel when you get there, and state it in the present tense as if it has already happened:

> *It is now 31st October 2012 and I feel so peaceful, connected and contented around my food choices that it is like living a different life. I no longer suffer inner battles with myself. I feel good about everything that I eat. And these food-related choices have enabled me to deepen the relationship I have with myself and to the planet as a whole, as I now feel a reverence for everything that I am blessed to be surrounded by. By working with my Type I have found a way to achieve this goal without any sense of 'loss' or deprivation. As a peaceful eater I feel as if I have discovered an amazing secret to living in a way that is so much deeper and richer than any I have ever discovered before. I am so glad that I made the shifts I made to get here. It has taken some effort, but my goodness the rewards have been abundant and inspiring; every day I feel increasingly better about this move. I feel humbled.*

Put It Up

Put your SMART goal somewhere you can see it every day, multiple times per day. Consider making more than one copy so that you can carry one in your wallet or purse.

Visualize It

See yourself – inside and out – feeling genuinely happy, peaceful and connected to everything you eat. Feel how it would be to feel truly happy about everything you put into your body and how that affects the way you look, think, feel and act. Allow yourself to enjoy this Possibility and know that you have the power and tools that you need to create this reality for yourself. It is a 'road less travelled', but a wonderfully rewarding one that will change every aspect of your life.

Commit to It

Commit to giving yourself this Possibility – in a way that works for you. Know that by working with your type and engaging heart and soul, you can start creating this reality from this moment forward.

Action Steps

What follows are three powerful action steps per Eater Type that will help you to enjoy your food more in a way that is a good fit for you. If your current eating style is a combination of more than one Type, simply read the action steps for each Type and decide which action steps are going to work best for you. If you'd like to integrate action steps from other Types in order to try on a new Eater Type profile to reach your specific eating for peace, connection and contentment goals, that's absolutely fine. However, do be clear that your main consideration is to be completely honest about what you *know* will work for you, taking into account what you know about yourself, what resonates for you when you read about each Type, and how you have experienced your behaviour when you've chosen to eat and drink with abandon before.

Get a pen and paper to finalize your unique list of action steps. There is a Menu Plan template at the back of this book, or you can also download it for free (together with a special action steps sheet) at ERFYPTBonuses.com, to make the process super-easy and fun.

The Functional Eater

You need a peace, connection and contentment plan that is quick and easy to follow and that involves minimum fuss, tastes delicious and helps you to reach your peace, connection and contentment goals simply and easily.

Your Three Best-fit Action Steps

1. List all the foods that you know automatically put you in touch with yourself and make you feel centred, calm and balanced, and that are quick and easy to prepare without sacrificing quality.

2. Create or find a menu plan that revolves around these foods and drinks while taking on the intention to eat in a way that is peaceful, connected and contented.

3. Make three copies of your plan: one for your kitchen, one for your bedroom, one for your wallet or purse. Make sure you stick to it.

The Sensual Eater

You need a peace, connection and contentment plan that satisfies all your senses, is just as pleasurable (or more so) as your usual menu to eat, and enables you to reach your peace, connection and contentment goals deliciously and decadently.

Your Three Best-fit Action Steps

1. Buy some new chinaware, glassware or anything for your kitchen that can be used as part of a new nurturing and supportive ritual.

2. Create or find a menu plan that delights you, where everything on your menu feels like a 10/10 for you, while at the same time creates a truly sacred experience with

food for you, because of the time and attention put into creating this plan.

3. Find sensual and nurturing ways to reward and indulge yourself that are non-edible, to complement the food choices you are making as you journey along this special path.

The Intellectual Eater

You need a peace, connection and contentment plan that makes complete sense to you, with no questions left unanswered and that 'adds up' in your head to help you matter-of-factly reach your peace, connection and contentment goals.

Your Three Best-fit Action Steps

1. List 10 compelling reasons why you want to become more peaceful, connected and contented.

2. Create or find a menu plan that comprises clean, non- or low-processed foods that keep you balanced and calm while meeting your other needs.

3. List 10 different ways that you know peace, connection and contentment could/do show up for you, and tick each one off once you experience it.

The Emotional Eater

You need a peace, connection and contentment plan that allows you to continue to use food in a way that nurtures you but using foods that enable you to reach your peace, connection and contentment goals comfortably.

Your Three Best-fit Action Steps

1. List 10 different non-edible treats that you know will make you feel more peaceful, connected and contented.

Whenever you find yourself wanting to eat when not hungry, pick one of these treats and enjoy.

2. Create or find a menu plan that incorporates the comfort foods and other foods that you know will make you feel more peaceful, connected and contented, but that do not damage you or your other goals in any way.

3. Consider meditating daily for 15 minutes and/or spending 15 minutes daily writing in a journal, processing your feelings about your day and how you are experiencing food and emotions differently through this new approach/focus.

The Focused Eater

You need a peace, connection and contentment plan that is to-the-point, easy to follow, that is clearly going to work and enables you to reach your peace, connection and contentment goals efficiently and enjoyably.

Your Three Best-fit Action Steps

1. List 15 different ways that you want peace, connection and contentment to show up for you, and tick each one off once you experience it (and sustain it).

2. Create or find a menu plan that you feel confident will get you the results you seek.

3. Invest in whatever tools, support or equipment you need to help you reach your peace, connection and contentment goals successfully.

The Intuitive Eater

You need a peace, connection and contentment plan that feels a great fit for you, enables you some flexibility depending on your hunger levels, and enables you to reach your peace, connection and contentment goals sensitively.

Your Three Best-fit Action Steps

1. Make a list of foods that you know for sure bring or sustain the feelings of peace, connection and contentment for you.

2. Create or find a menu plan that comprises these foods and any others that you are drawn to when you set the intention to eat for this experience.

3. Pay attention to your energetic reaction to each food or ingredient you eat as you follow your menu plan; tweak accordingly until you reach the level of peace, connection and contentment that you desire.

The Conscious Eater

You need a peace, connection and contentment plan that satisfies your soul, is a perfect fit for your highest philosophy, and enables you to reach your peace, connection and contentment goals easily and peacefully.

Your Three Best-fit Action Steps

1. Make a list of all the foods that you know bring you the most peace, connection and contentment *and* fit in perfectly with your personal food philosophy.

2. Create or find a menu plan that orientates itself around these foods and any others that work for you on these important levels.

3. Integrate your eating habits with any other complementary practices that you know will support and maximize this experience, such as tai chi, yoga, meditation or journaling.

The Experimental Eater

You need a peace, connection and contentment plan that is as varied as you love things to be, introduces you to new and exciting foods, and allows you to reach your peace, connection and contentment goals creatively and enthusiastically.

Your Three Best-fit Action Steps

1. Make a list of all the foods that are purported to bring greater levels of peace, connection and contentment to the body.

2. Create or find a menu plan that incorporates these foods, together with any others you enjoy and which you already know bring you greater levels of peace, connection and contentment. Make sure your final menu plan feels really exciting to you – but in a non-stimulating way!

3. Determine how and where you're going to get the new foods, and create a plan that enables this to happen easily and joyfully.

The Confused Eater

You need a peace, connection and contentment plan that makes total sense to you, raises no questions whatsoever, and that enables you to reach your peace, connection and contentment goals confidently and purposefully.

Your Three Best-fit Action Steps

1. Write a list of all the foods and drinks you absolutely KNOW are going to help you feel more peaceful, connected and contented, and also that you enjoy.

2. Create or find a menu plan that contains these foods – hire a nutritionist or professional healthcare provider to make the plan for you if you feel this is important.

3. Make a commitment to follow this plan for *at least* three weeks – you can reformat your menu plan after that if you feel you want or need to.

The Social Eater

You need a peace, connection and contentment plan that is fun and flexible to follow, that allows you to socialize as much as you've always done, and that enables you to reach your peace, connection and contentment goals joyfully and playfully.

Your Three Best-fit Action Steps

1. Make a list of all the places or social gatherings you love to eat at, are soon to eat at, and want to eat at. Highlight the ones that you know will serve the most peace-, connection- and contentment-friendly foods.

2. Create a menu plan that incorporates these places, the meals you will eat while there, as well as the everyday-at-home foods that will enable you to experience the level of peace, connection and contentment that you seek.

3. Design and host a special dinner party or other food-centred event that supports your goal and revolves around the theme of 'peace, connection and contentment' (or any of these three qualities). Choose foods, activities and dress that embody this theme.

Now you've read about each type and the recommended action steps, it's time to write your unique list of action steps that you *know* will get you to your goal/s in a way that feels great to you.

My Unique Peace, Connection and Contented Eating Plan

Write down your peace, connection and contentment affirmation. Keep it with you and/or put it up somewhere you can see it every day. Example affirmation: 'Nothing brings me greater pleasure than to nourish my body in a way that makes me feel more peaceful, connected to and contented with my body, myself and others.'

Write down your specific 'I am going to love this' action steps.

Now you have your plan, it's time to put it into action.

You can do this! This is your own personal recipe for eating in a way that is holistically fulfilling and infinitely rewarding. Life will never be the same again!

EATING FOR OPTIMUM NUTRITION 🍎

There's no doubt about it, the more nutrient-dense our diet, the better we get to look, feel and perform. It is widely acknowledged that most people alive today, even in more affluent parts of the world, are suffering from some kind of nutritional deficiency. The impact of this can vary from low-level depression, malaise and lack of energy right through to full-on life-threatening illnesses.

Wherever you are at in your life and food journey, paying attention to what you eat is only ever going to be a good thing, but taking it to the level where you're proactively making sure that your diet is as abundant in nutrients as possible is something else entirely.

This Possibility is probably the best one for you if you know, instinctively or as a result of a diagnosis, that you would benefit from paying close attention to what you eat and learning to eat the most nutrient-rich diet for you.

Everyone would benefit from exploring and focusing on this Possibility at different stages throughout their lives. Perhaps this is the perfect time for you.

Eating for nutrition is for you if:

- You know that your diet could do with some serious improvement

- You like the idea of knowing exactly what you're putting into your body and how that will benefit you

- You are suffering from a deficiency and want to focus on correcting it

- You want to find out what would happen if you upped the level of nutrients in your diet

- You are not feeling your best and you want to take a measured, specific approach to looking and feeling better.

The Eater Types that you could run with or integrate for experiencing more nutrition with your food:

- **The Functional Eater** – will lessen any emotion that you feel around food which might otherwise hold you back from doing what needs to be done.

- **The Intellectual Eater** – will get super-excited about being able to sit down with a nutritionist, book or other resource to figure out the right dietary plan for you.

- **The Focused Eater** – will support you by setting specific nutritional profile goals and helping you follow the menu plan and action steps to get you into tip-top health.

- **The Intuitive Eater** – will help you on a sixth-sense level to know what to eat and when without having to refer to a textbook.

- **The Experimental Eater** – will help you get excited about trying new things and finding exotic herbs and superfoods to bump up your nutritional intake.

Using Your Dominant Type in a Way That Works

Get Clear

Get clear on your goal and write it down – make it a SMART goal, that is: Specific, Measurable, Achievable, Realistic and Timely. Also, imagine how you will look and feel when you get there, and state it in the present tense as if it has already happened:

It is now 31st October 2012 and I feel truly healthy and alive in my body. All of the niggling health issues that had been bothering me, all of the moments where I thought something was wrong, have dissipated. Now I wake up every day feeling happy and confident that I am doing the best by my body, and the results I have been seeing and feeling confirm that I am

*absolutely on the right track. By working with my Type/s I found
that it was easy for me to make the changes I needed to make.
It was actually joyful, rewarding and expansive. I am so glad that
I took the time and made the effort to educate myself on how my
body works and what foods are best for me to achieve optimum
health. I feel radiant!*

Put It Up

Put your SMART goal somewhere you can see it every day,
multiple times per day. Consider making more than one copy
so that you can carry one in your wallet or purse.

Visualize It

See yourself – inside and out – feeling strong, powerful and
firing on all cylinders. Feel how it would be to feel this alive
and 'tanked up'. Allow yourself to enjoy this Possibility and
know that with the right education and action this can be your
reality. Just think, also, that when you do this for yourself, how
many other people you can also help along the way.

Commit to It

Commit to giving yourself this Possibility – in a way that
works for you. Know that by embodying the types that get
excited about this mission, you can experience a level of
health and energy that you never dreamed existed.

Action Steps

What follows are three powerful action steps per Eater Type
that will help you to create the most nutritious eating plan
for you. If your current eating style is a combination of more
than one Type, simply read the action steps for each Type and
decide which ones are going to work best for you. If you'd

like to integrate action steps from other Types in order to try on a new Eater Type profile to reach your specific eating for nutrition goals, that's absolutely fine. However, do be clear that your main consideration is to be completely honest about what you *know* will work for you, taking into account what you know about yourself, what resonates for you when you read about each Type, and how much you have focused on eating for nutrition in the past.

Get a pen and paper to finalize your unique list of action steps. There is a Menu Plan template at the back of this book, or you can also download it for free (together with a special action steps sheet) at ERFYPTBonuses.com, to make the process super-easy and fun.

The Functional Eater

You need a nutrition plan that is quick and easy to follow and that involves minimum fuss, tastes delicious and helps you to reach your nutrition goals simply and easily.

Your Three Best-fit Action Steps

1. Buy, borrow or find a book on top-level nutrition and/or superfoods, and list all the foods you want to eat that will supercharge your nutritional intake. Also make note of where you can get them (ideally pre-made) to make this really easy for you. Next, list the mail order companies, local takeaways and other super-easy-to-use services that will give you exactly what you want with minimal input on your part.

2. Create or find a menu plan that is quick, easy and delicious to follow, that incorporates these foods and drinks wherever possible, and includes other meals that you can quickly pull together yourself (in 10 minutes or less) that will help you reach your nutrition goals.

3. Make three copies of your plan: one for your kitchen, one for your bedroom, one for your wallet or purse. Make sure you stick to it.

The Sensual Eater

You need a nutrition plan that satisfies all your senses, is just as pleasurable as your usual menu to eat (or even more so) and that enables you to reach your nutrition goals deliciously and decadently.

Your Three Best-fit Action Steps

1. Buy, borrow or find a book on top-level nutrition and/ or superfoods, and list all the foods that look or sound enjoyable, decadent and exciting to you *and* that will supercharge your nutritional intake.

2. Create or find a menu plan that excites you, where everything on your menu feels like a 10/10 for you, and where your desires are being met through super-nutritious foods and drinks.

3. Find sensual ways to reward and indulge yourself that are non-edible as you reach nutrition goals along the way to your final destination.

The Intellectual Eater

You need a nutrition plan that makes complete sense to you, with no questions left unanswered and that 'adds up' in your head to help you matter-of-factly reach your nutrition goals.

Your Three Best-fit Action Steps

1. List 10 compelling reasons why upping the level of nutrition in your diet will benefit you.

2. Create or find a menu plan that adds up in a way that makes sense to you, in order to take the amount of nutrition in your diet to its highest ever level.

3. Set nutrition-related goals that feel realistic and achievable according to weekly time-frames, and create a chart where you can keep track of your progress.

The Emotional Eater

You need a nutrition plan that allows you to continue to use food in a way that nurtures you but using foods that enable you to reach your nutrition goals comfortably.

Your Three Best-fit Action Steps

1. Buy, borrow or find a book on top-level nutrition and/ or superfoods, and list all the foods that look or sound enjoyable, decadent and comforting to you *and* that will supercharge your nutritional intake.

2. Create or find a menu plan that revolves around these highly nutritious foods as well as super-healthy versions of the comfort foods you are used to reaching for.

3. Work with a nutritionist or professional healthcare provider to help you create this plan and/or maintain it so that you have professional input as you make this transition.

The Focused Eater

You need a nutrition plan that is to-the-point, easy to follow, that is clearly going to work and enables you to reach your nutrition goals efficiently and enjoyably.

Your Three Best-fit Action Steps

1. Create a nutrient-tracker that clearly maps out your ultimate dietary goal and your smaller incremental

goals so you can check against them daily/weekly as appropriate.

2. Create or find a menu plan that you feel confident will deliver the amount of nutrition that you seek.

3. Invest in whatever tools, support or equipment you need to help you reach your nutrition goal/s successfully.

The Intuitive Eater

You need a nutrition plan that feels a great fit for you, enables you some flexibility depending on your hunger levels, and enables you to reach your nutrition goals sensitively.

Your Three Best-fit Action Steps

1. Buy, borrow or find a book on top-level nutrition and/or superfoods and list all the foods that will supercharge your nutritional intake and that you know your body always responds well to. Also consider other foods that you haven't tried before.

2. Create or find a menu plan that comprises these foods and that will also lead to your nutritional goal/s being met.

3. Pay close attention to how you feel on various different levels as you follow your menu plan; tweak it accordingly until you reach your nutrition goals and feel great about what you're eating.

The Conscious Eater

You need a nutrition plan that satisfies your soul, is a perfect fit for your highest philosophy, and enables you to reach your nutrition goals easily and peacefully.

Your Three Best-fit Action Steps

1. Buy, borrow or find a book on top-level nutrition and/or superfoods and list all the foods that are a great fit for your personal philosophy and that will impart the greatest levels of nutrition to your body.

2. Create or find a menu plan that revolves around these foods and that makes you feel good on every level.

3. Keep a running list of all the ways your body and energy (and anything else that's important to you) change and benefit from your nutritional advances as you go.

The Experimental Eater

You need a nutrition plan that is as varied as you love things to be, introduces you to new and exciting foods, and allows you to reach your nutrition goals creatively and enthusiastically.

Your Three Best-fit Action Steps

1. Buy, borrow or find a book on top-level nutrition and/or superfoods; make a list of all the foods you'd love to try but haven't yet that are cited as high-nutrient foods.

2. Create or find a menu plan that incorporates these foods in abundance, together with your regular high-nutrient favourites. Make sure your final menu plan feels really exciting to you.

3. Determine how and where you're going to get these foods; create a plan that enables this to happen easily and joyfully.

The Confused Eater

You need a nutrition plan that makes total sense to you, raises no questions whatsoever, and that enables you to reach your nutrition goals confidently and purposefully.

Your Three Best-fit Action Steps

1. Buy, borrow or find a book on top-level nutrition and/or superfoods, and compile a list of all the foods and drinks you absolutely KNOW and believe are going to help you to up your nutrient-intake significantly, to the level you desire, and that you will enjoy.

2. Create or find a menu plan that contains these foods – hire a nutritionist or professional healthcare provider to make the plan for you if you feel you could benefit from this.

3. Make a commitment to follow this plan for at least four weeks – you can reformat your menu plan after that if you feel you want or need to.

The Social Eater

You need a nutrition plan that is fun and flexible to follow, that allows you to socialize as much as you've always done, and that enables you to reach your nutrition goals joyfully and playfully.

Your Three Best-fit Action Steps

1. Buy, borrow or find a book on top-level nutrition and/ or superfoods and make a list of all the places or social gatherings you love to eat at, are soon to eat at, and could eat at that would serve especially nutrient-dense meals.

2. Create a menu plan that incorporates these places, the meals you will eat while there as well as the everyday-at-home high-nutrient foods you like to eat.

3. Host a special dinner party or other social gathering where all the foods and drinks served are nutrient-dense so you can have fun while exploring new ingredients and recipes with your friends.

Now you've read about each type and the recommended action steps, it's time to write your unique list of action steps that you *know* will get you to your goal/s in a way that feels great to you.

My Unique Eating for Nutrition Plan

Write down your eating for nutrition affirmation. Keep it with you and/or put it up somewhere you can see it every day. Example affirmation: 'By feeding my body the very best, most nutritious foods, I am telling myself that I count, I matter and I am worth all of this and more.'

Now write down your specific 'I am going to love this' action steps.

Now you have your plan, it's time to put it into action.

You can do this! This is your own personal recipe for recreating your body using only the finest ingredients. Use the vision of the new, powered-up you as continual inspiration for this rewarding path ahead.

EATING FOR SELF-KNOWLEDGE 🍎

The concept of eating for self-knowledge might seem a strange one, but it's actually a phenomenal tool for personal and spiritual growth. This is because what you eat, as you have already learned, says so much about you that's it's a fantastic mirror for showing you exactly who you are, and exactly where you're at. What's also great about food as a tool for self-awareness is that it will clearly show you the gap between what you intellectually or intuitively know and how much of that you are actually applying in your life. It's in this gap that you get to see what needs to happen for you to be 'walking the walk' or, at the very least, taking your knowledge and using it to put you in a place of whole-person integrity, honesty and alignment.

This Possibility is the one to choose if you are ready for some serious introspection and personal growth. Beyond this point you can refine and hone your diet to your heart's content, but at this stage you can gain a whole level of awareness that no other Possibility, with the exception Eating For Peace, Connection and Contentment, can even come close to. This is manna from heaven for those who love to know who they are and what they're about.

Eating for self-knowledge is for you if:

- You know that there's a gap between what you know you 'should' be eating and what you actually are eating

- You want to use food and eating as tools for awareness and insight into yourself

- You are fascinated to see what will be revealed to you as you delve into the world of self-enquiry through food

- You want to choose a food path that is a perfect fit for who you want to become

- You are ready to face many truths about yourself, no matter how they may show up.

The Eater Types that you could run with or integrate for experiencing greater self-knowledge:

- **The Functional Eater** – will enable you to eat very simply and for hunger alone in order to reveal to you those times when you eat for any other reasons.

- **The Sensual Eater** – will enable you to delve into discovering what brings you pleasure, and how you could bring more of that into the rest of your life (and not just through food!).

- **The Intuitive Eater** – will help you tune in to what foods and eating 'path' are naturally right for you as an individual, free of dogma and limiting labels.

- **The Conscious Eater** – will put you through the fire of compassion by helping you see to what extent you feel comfortable consuming foods and drinks that have caused pain, suffering or destruction on their journey to your table.

- **The Experimental Eater** – will open you up to new ways of looking at food and consuming it, just to see what does and doesn't work for you on different levels.

- **The Social Eater** – will flag up to you how much of your eating is dictated by your need to please, fit in or be seen as somebody that you're truly not.

Using Your Dominant Type in a Way That Works

Get Clear

Get clear on your goal and write it down – make it a SMART goal, that is: Specific, Measurable, Achievable, Realistic and Timely. Also, imagine how you will look and feel when you get there, and state it in the present tense as if it has already happened:

It is now 31st October 2012 and I am feeling blown away by the level of congruency that I am now living and enjoying. Through doing this process I learned that there were so many different ways that I was undermining the truth of who I am. Now I know exactly who I am and what I stand for and why. I choose to eat the way that I eat and am totally clear on why I'm doing it. By working with my Type/s I had a ball spending time learning more about myself through the medium of food. I knew that it would be interesting, but I didn't expect to learn as much as I really did learn. Now my whole life and every moment is benefiting. I am in awe!

Put It Up

Put your SMART goal somewhere you can see it every day, multiple times per day. Consider making more than one copy so that you can carry one in your wallet or purse.

Visualize It

See yourself – inside and out – feeling strong, powerful and firing on all cylinders. Feel how it would be to feel this alive and 'tanked up'. Allow yourself to enjoy this Possibility and know that with the right education and action this can be your reality. Just think also that when you do this for yourself, how many other people you can also help along the way.

Commit to It

Commit to giving yourself this Possibility – in a way that works for you. By starting with what you know to be true you will be on a much faster track to revealing the total picture.

Action Steps

What follows are three powerful action steps per Eater Type that will help you to create the most self-revealing eating plan for you. If your current eating style is a combination of more than one Type, simply read the action steps for each Type and decide which action steps are going to work best for you. If you'd like to integrate action steps from other Types in order to try on a new Eater Type profile to reach your specific eating for self-knowledge goals, that's absolutely fine. However, do be clear that your main consideration is to be completely honest about what you *know* will work for you, taking into account what you know about yourself, what resonates for you when you read about each Type, and how you much you have focused on eating for self-discovery/self-knowledge in the past.

Get a pen and paper to finalize your unique list of action steps. There is a Menu Plan template at the back of this book, or you can also download it for free (together with a special action steps sheet) at ERFYPTBonuses.com, to make the process super-easy and fun.

The Functional Eater

You need a self-knowledge plan that is quick and easy to follow and that involves minimum fuss, tastes delicious and helps you to reach your self-knowledge goals simply and easily.

Your Three Best-fit Action Steps

1. List all the foods that you eat on a regular basis. Next to each one write a single word or sentence that best describes what you know to be true about each food (e.g. coffee = stimulating; wheat = makes me gain weight; chocolate = I don't really want or need it).

2. Create or find a menu plan that is quick, easy and delicious to follow, which incorporates only the foods that you know you like and that you can feel truly good about eating.

3. Make three copies of your plan: one for your kitchen, one for your bedroom, one for your wallet or purse; make sure you stick to it. Pay attention to what awarenesses come up for you if and when you find yourself straying from the menu plan. What are your choices telling you? What are you learning about yourself?

The Sensual Eater

You need a self-knowledge plan that satisfies all your senses, is just as pleasurable as your usual menu to eat (or more) and that enables you to reach your self-knowledge goals deliciously and decadently.

Your Three Best-fit Action Steps

1. List all the foods that you eat on a regular basis, as well as the ones you find yourself reaching for when eating out. Next to each one write a single word or sentence that best describes what you know to be true about each food (e.g. coffee = stimulating; wheat = makes me gain weight; chocolate = I don't really want or need it).

2. Create or find a menu plan that excites you, where everything on your menu feels like a 10/10 for you – that means you love it, but you also know that it loves you.

3. Pay attention to any awarenesses that come up for you if and when you find yourself straying from your menu plan. What are your choices telling you? What are you learning about yourself?

The Intellectual Eater

You need a self-knowledge plan that makes complete sense to you, with no questions left unanswered and that 'adds up' in your head to help you matter-of-factly reach your self-knowledge goals.

Your Three Best-fit Action Steps

1. List 10 compelling reasons why you want to gain greater self-knowledge and how that will benefit you.

2. List all the foods that you tend towards eating on a day-to-day basis, and next to each one write a single word or sentence that best describes what you know to be true about each food (e.g. coffee = stimulating; wheat = makes me gain weight; chocolate = I don't really want or need it).

3. Create or find a menu plan that comprises only the foods and drinks that you know are a perfect fit for you on every level. Pay attention to what awarenesses come up for you if and when you find yourself straying from the menu plan. What are your choices telling you? What are you learning about yourself?

The Emotional Eater

You need a self-knowledge plan that allows you to continue to use food in a way that nurtures you but using foods that enable you to reach your self-knowledge goals comfortably.

Your Three Best-fit Action Steps

1. List 10 compelling reasons why you want to gain greater self-knowledge and how that will benefit you.

2. List all the foods that you tend towards eating on a day-to-day basis, and next to each one write a single word or sentence that best describes what you know to be true about each food (e.g. coffee = stimulating; wheat = makes me gain weight; chocolate = I don't really want or need it).

3. Create or find a menu plan that comprises only the foods and drinks that you know are a perfect fit for you on every level. Pay attention to awarenesses that come up for you if and when you find yourself straying from the menu plan.

What are your choices telling you? What are you learning about yourself? Journal for 15 minutes per day in order to process what you are learning. Seek professional support if what you are learning about yourself is something you need counselling or therapy around.

The Focused Eater

You need a self-knowledge plan that is to-the-point, easy to follow, that is clearly going to work and enables you to reach your self-knowledge goals efficiently and enjoyably.

Your Three Best-fit Action Steps

1. List 10 ways you will know you have learned what you wanted to learn about yourself through this eating approach, so you can check off the list as you reach each milestone.

2. Create or find a menu plan that comprises foods and drinks that you know will give you 'nowhere to run and nowhere to hide' on every level, so you can receive quick and insightful feedback from what happens when you try to follow the plan. Pay attention to what awarenesses come up for you if and when you find yourself straying from the menu plan. What are your choices telling you? What are you learning about yourself?

3. Invest in whatever tools, support or equipment you need to help you learn even more about yourself as you commit to garnering deeper self-knowledge.

The Intuitive Eater

You need a self-knowledge plan that feels a great fit for you, enables you some flexibility depending on your hunger levels, and enables you to reach your self-knowledge goals sensitively.

Your Three Best-fit Action Steps

1. Make a list of foods that your body has been asking for recently and today; analyse each one according to what you know to be true about what those foods do to or for you (e.g. ice-cream = comforts me; bread = relaxes me; cheese = nourishes me).

2. Create or find a menu plan that comprises foods that you know you are 'into' at the moment and that you feel good about on every level – that is, ones that you know are not damaging, stifling or comforting in any way.

3. Pay attention to what awarenesses come up for you if and when you find yourself straying from the menu plan. What are your choices telling you? What are you learning about yourself?

The Conscious Eater

You need a self-knowledge plan that satisfies your soul, is a perfect fit for your highest philosophy, and enables you to reach your self-knowledge goals easily and peacefully.

Your Three Best-fit Action Steps

1. List 10 soulful reasons why you want to gain greater self-knowledge at this point in your life.

2. List all the foods that you tend towards eating on a day-to-day basis, and next to each one write a single word or sentence that best describes what you know to be true about each food (e.g. coffee = stimulating; wheat = makes me gain weight; chocolate = I don't really want or need it).

3. Create or find a menu plan made up of only those foods and drinks that you know are a perfect fit for you on every level. Pay attention to what awarenesses come up for you if and when you find yourself straying from the menu plan. What are your choices telling you? What are you learning

about yourself? Journal for 15 minutes a day in order to process what you are learning, and/or meditate on what's happening to gain even greater awareness and insight.

The Experimental Eater

You need a self-knowledge plan that is as varied as you love things to be, introduces you to new and exciting foods, and allows you to reach your self-knowledge goals creatively and enthusiastically.

Your Three Best-fit Action Steps

1. Make a list of all the foods that you've been wanting to try and have on your mental 'hit list', as well as the five most recent new foods that you've tried. Next to each one write a single word or sentence that best describes what you know or believe to be true about each of these foods (e.g. durian = aphrodisiac; jackfruit = juicy; raw cacao bean = stimulating).

2. Looking at your list of foods and words, what are your choices telling you? What are you learning about yourself? If you look closely you will see patterns and themes that are mirroring back to you what's important in your life right now.

3. Go about your eating as normal, but for the next three weeks pay really close attention to what you are reaching for. As you go to eat or order each food (or drink), ask yourself, 'What is the promise I believe this food holds for me?' (e.g. happiness, comfort, excitement, mystery) and see what it is you are trying to buy into.

The Confused Eater

You need a self-knowledge plan that makes total sense to you, raises no questions whatsoever, and that enables you to reach your self-knowledge goals confidently and purposefully.

Your Three Best-fit Action Steps

1. List 10 compelling reasons why you want to gain greater self-knowledge, and how that will benefit you.

2. List all the foods that you tend towards eating on a day-to-day basis, and next to each one write a single word or sentence that best describes what you know to be true about each food (e.g. coffee = stimulating; wheat = makes me gain weight; chocolate = I don't really want or need it).

3. Create or find a menu plan that comprises only the foods and drinks that you *know* are a perfect fit for you on every level. Pay attention to what awarenesses come up for you if and when you find yourself straying from the menu plan. What are your choices telling you? What are you learning about yourself? Make a commitment with yourself to follow this plan for at *least* three weeks – you can reformat your menu plan after that if you feel you want or need to.

The Social Eater

You need a self-knowledge plan that is fun and flexible to follow, that allows you to socialize as much as you've always done, and that enables you to reach your self-knowledge goals joyfully and playfully.

Your Three Best-fit Action Steps

1. Make a list of all your favourite foods, drinks and restaurants. Next to each one write a single word or sentence that best describes what you know or believe to be true about each of them or what you feel they 'give' to you (e.g. wine = happiness; soup = comfort; 'Simon's Place' = belonging.)

2. Looking at your list of foods, eateries and words, what are your choices telling you? What are you learning about yourself? If you look closely you will see patterns and

themes that are mirroring back to you what's important and what's going on in your life right now.

3. Go about your eating as normal, but for the next three weeks pay really close attention to what you are reaching for. As you go to eat or order each food (or drink), ask yourself, 'What is the promise I believe this food holds for me?' (e.g. happiness, comfort, excitement, mystery). Do the same for your choice of eating establishments. And from all the insights you gather, see what it is you are trying to buy into.

Now you've read about each type and the recommended action steps, it's time to write your unique list of action steps that you *know* will get you to your goal/s in a way that feels great to you.

My Unique Eating for Self-knowledge Plan

Write down your eating for self-knowledge affirmation. Keep it with you and/or put it up somewhere you can see it every day. Example affirmation: 'The more I pay attention to what I want to eat, the more I learn about myself and what I truly want for myself at this point in my life.'

Now write down your specific 'I am going to love this' action steps.

Now you have your plan, it's time to put it into action.

You can do this! This is your own personal recipe for creating a space to get to truly see and understand yourself. Go on, be brave, the best is yet to come…

EATING FOR COMFORT 🍎

Everyone knows what it is to eat for comfort, even if they might not know when they are doing it. In fact, so common is this behaviour that the term 'comfort-eating' is one that everyone has heard of and has probably used on more than one occasion in their lives to describe their own behaviour.

It's not wrong to comfort-eat; it's just not the most appropriate use for food. And of course it never solves any problem – in fact, it often compounds them. Nonetheless it does tend to work on some level – that level being where raw emotion is felt and eating is the perfect antidote to experiencing that. It can numb the pain long enough to move to a better moment, like sleep or work or being busy, but it can never, ever take it away.

So why would we *choose* to eat for comfort? Because if you're going to do it, then do it consciously, I say. Because there's no doubt that there are always going to be times in life when, despite knowing that there are healthier ways of handling emotions, all that we're really capable of in that moment is spooning into something cool and creamy, or deftly removing a cork from a bottle of red. With this being a very real possibility, it makes sense to find alternative ways of handling these times so that, if and when they do arise, you handle them in a way that feels loving rather than abusive.

This Possibility is the one to choose if you are going through a difficult time in your life right now or know that you are prone to times like this. It's also a great Possibility to explore if you want to build in a little 'wriggle room' in an otherwise high-maintenance diet.

Eating for comfort is for you if:

- You are going through a tough time right now and want to handle it sanely

- You know you have a predisposal to eating for comfort and want to find healthier ways to do it when you do

- You want to build in some 'comfort' to any existing diet plan so you can relax when you want to without guilt

- You want to have a strategy in place for eating for comfort, just in case you need to.

The Eater Types that you could run with or integrate for experiencing greater comfort:

- **The Sensual Eater** – will enable you to explore and be honest about what foods have what effect on you so you can make effective choices.

- **The Focused Eater** – will help you create some supporting rules around your comfort-eating so it never escalates or deteriorates into a full-blown binge session.

- **The Social Eater** – will get you out into the world socializing so that you can find comfort and healing through good conversation with friends and loved ones.

Using Your Dominant Type in a Way That Works

Get Clear

Get clear on your goal and write it down – make it a SMART goal, that is: Specific, Measurable, Achievable, Realistic and Timely. Also, imagine how you will look and feel when you get there, and state it in the present tense as if it has already happened:

> It is now 31st October 2012 and I finally have a great relationship with food. In the past when I felt down I would automatically reach for a bag of crisps or a tub of Ben and Jerry's, but now I know how to handle myself and my emotions in a way that feels genuinely comforting – with or without food.

By working with my Type/s I came to create my own special way of being with food that nurtured me and supported me rather than letting myself become a victim of my own behaviour. I didn't think this was possible before, but now I know first-hand that when you take a big step back and put self-love first, eating for comfort in a sane and healthy way can actually become a reality. I am amazed!

Put It Up

Put your SMART goal somewhere you can see it every day, multiple times per day. Consider making more than one copy so that you can carry one in your wallet or purse.

Visualize It

See yourself – inside and out – feeling comforted, loved and secure whether you choose to comfort-eat food or not. Feel how it would be to love yourself enough to make the healthiest decision, even during the toughest times. Allow yourself to enjoy this Possibility and know that by putting yourself first you can create this gentle loving relationship between yourself and food.

Commit to It

Commit to giving yourself this Possibility – in a way that works for you. Your feelings and the way you express them are powerful and unique. Give yourself the gift of honouring this through the way you learn how to comfort yourself.

Action Steps

What follows are three powerful action steps per Eater Type that will help you to create the most comforting eating plan for you. If your current eating style is a combination of more than one Type, simply read the action steps for each Type and decide which action steps are going to work best for you. If you'd like to integrate action steps from other Types in order to try on a new Eater Type profile to create your specific eating for comfort plan/guidelines, that's absolutely fine. However, do be clear that your main consideration is to be rigorously honest, taking into account what you know about yourself, what resonates for you when you read about each Type, and how much you have mastered 'sane' comfort-eating in the past.

Get a pen and paper to finalize your unique list of action steps. There is a Menu Plan template at the back of this book, or you can also download it for free (together with a special action steps sheet) at ERFYPTBonuses.com, to make the process super-easy and fun.

The Functional Eater

You need a comfort plan that is quick and easy to follow and that involves minimum fuss, tastes delicious and helps you to reach your comfort goals simply and easily.

Your Three Best-fit Action Steps

1. List all the foods and drinks that you love to consume and that you know genuinely do bring you comfort on some level when you have them. Next, list the mail order companies, local takeaways and other super-easy-to-use services that will give you exactly what you want, when the time arises, with minimal input on your part.

2. Where possible, pre-buy in these foods and drinks so they are there for you if you want them, but – most importantly – set 'healthy' parameters for yourself about what your 'one-sitting limit' is for each of these items so you can eat them when you want to, but *not* go over the top.

3. Decide and act on one complementary therapy, practice or habit that will soothe you emotionally during this emotional time, or obtain professional counselling if necessary.

The Sensual Eater

You need a comfort plan that satisfies all your senses, is just as pleasurable as your usual menu to eat (or more) and that enables you to reach your comfort goals deliciously and decadently.

Your Three Best-fit Action Steps

1. Buy some new chinaware, glassware or anything that you eat or drink from that delights and inspires you. You will use this to eat or drink from when you eat for comfort. This way you get to treat comfort-eating as nourishment for your soul rather than something self-harming.

2. List all the foods and drinks that you love to consume which you know genuinely do bring you comfort on some level when you have them. Where possible, pre-buy in these foods so they are there for you if you want them, but – most importantly – set 'healthy' parameters for yourself about what your 'one-sitting limit' is for each of these foods so you can eat them when you want to but not go over the top.

3. Decide and act on one to three complementary therapies, practices or habits that will soothe you emotionally during this time, or obtain professional counselling if necessary.

The Intellectual Eater

You need a comfort plan that makes complete sense to you, with no questions left unanswered and that 'adds up' in your head to help you matter-of-factly reach your comfort goals.

Your Three Best-fit Action Steps

1. List 10 reasons why you feel the need to eat for comfort right now.

2. List all the foods and drinks that you know genuinely do bring you comfort on some level when you have them, but also that you don't feel terribly bad about eating. Where possible, pre-buy in these foods and drinks so they are there for you if you want them, but – most importantly – set 'healthy' parameters for yourself about what your 'one-sitting limit' is for each of these items so you can eat them when you want to, but *not* go over the top.

3. Decide and act on one to three complementary therapies, practices or habits that will soothe you during this emotional time, or obtain professional counselling if necessary.

The Emotional Eater

You need a comfort plan that allows you to continue to use food in a way that nurtures you but using foods that enable you to reach your comfort goals comfortably.

Your Three Best-fit Action Steps

1. List all the different reasons why you feel the need to eat for comfort right now and secure the appropriate support for helping you to overcome the issues which are troubling you.

2. List 10 different non-edible treats that you know will 'fill you up' emotionally. Whenever you find yourself wanting to eat for emotion, indulge in one of these instead of food or drink wherever possible.

3. List all the foods and drinks that you know genuinely do bring you comfort on some level when you have them, but

also that you don't feel terribly bad about eating. Where possible, pre-buy in these foods and drinks so they are there for you if you want them, but – most importantly – set 'healthy' parameters for yourself about what your 'one-sitting limit' is for each of these items so you can eat them when you want to, but *not* go over the top.

The Focused Eater

You need a comfort plan that is to-the-point, easy to follow, that is clearly going to work and enables you to reach your comfort goals efficiently and enjoyably.

Your Three Best-fit Action Steps

1. List all of the reasons why you feel the need to eat for comfort right now.

2. List all the foods and drinks that you know genuinely do bring you comfort on some level when you have them, but that you feel great about eating. Where possible, pre-buy in these foods and drinks so they are there for you if you want them, but – most importantly – set 'healthy' parameters for yourself about what your 'one-sitting limit' is for each of these items so you can eat them when you want to, but *not* go over the top.

3. Decide and act on one to three complementary therapies, practices or habits that will soothe you during this emotional time, or obtain professional counselling if necessary.

The Intuitive Eater

You need a comfort plan that feels a great fit for you, enables you some flexibility depending on your hunger levels, and helps you to reach your comfort goals sensitively.

Your Three Best-fit Action Steps

1. List all of the reasons why you feel the need to eat for comfort right now.

2. List all the foods and drinks that you know genuinely do bring you comfort on some level when you have them, but that you still feel are intuitive choices. Where possible, pre-buy in these foods and drinks so they are there for you if you want them, but – most importantly – set 'healthy' parameters for yourself about what your 'one-sitting limit' is for each of these items so you can eat them when you want to, but *not* go over the top.

3. Decide and act on one to three complementary therapies, practices or habits that will soothe you during this emotional time, or obtain professional counselling if necessary.

The Conscious Eater

You need a comfort plan that satisfies your soul, is a perfect fit for your highest philosophy, and enables you to reach your comfort goals easily and peacefully.

Your Three Best-fit Action Steps

1. List all of the reasons why you feel the need to eat for comfort right now, and journal about each one if you have the time and inclination to do so (recommended).

2. List all the foods and drinks that you know genuinely do bring you comfort on some level when you have them, but that you still feel are conscious choices. Where possible, pre-buy in these foods and drinks so they are there for you if you want them, but – most importantly – set 'healthy' parameters for yourself about what your 'one-sitting limit' is for each of these items so you can eat them when you want to, but *not* go over the top.

3. Decide and act on one to three complementary therapies, practices or habits that will soothe you during this emotional time, or obtain professional counselling if necessary.

The Experimental Eater

You need a comfort plan that is as varied as you love things to be, introduces you to new and exciting foods, and allows you to reach your comfort goals creatively and enthusiastically.

Your Three Best-fit Action Steps

1. List all the reasons why you feel the need to eat for comfort right now.

2. List all the foods and drinks that you know genuinely do bring you comfort on some level when you have them, and be open to new ones that you might not have tried before. Where possible, pre-buy in these foods and drinks so they are there for you if you want them, but – most importantly – set 'healthy' parameters for yourself about what your 'one-sitting limit' is for each of these items so you can eat them when you want to, but *not* go over the top.

3. Decide and act on one to three complementary therapies, practices or habits that will soothe you during this emotional time, or obtain professional counselling if necessary.

The Confused Eater

You need a comfort plan that makes total sense to you, raises no questions whatsoever, and that enables you to reach your comfort goals confidently and purposefully.

Your Three Best-fit Action Steps

1. List all the reasons why you feel the need to eat for comfort right now.

2. List all the foods and drinks that you know genuinely do bring you comfort on some level when you have them, but that are basic and won't mess with your mind. Where possible, pre-buy in these foods and drinks so they are there for you if you want them, but – most importantly – set 'healthy' parameters for yourself about what your 'one-sitting limit' is for each of these items so you can eat them when you want to, but *not* go over the top.

3. Decide and act on one to three complementary therapies, practices or habits that will soothe you during this emotional time, or obtain professional counselling if necessary.

The Social Eater

You need a comfort plan that is fun and flexible to follow, that allows you to socialize as much as you've always done, and that enables you to reach your comfort goals joyfully and playfully.

Your Three Best-fit Action Steps

1. List all of the reasons why you feel the need to eat for comfort right now.

2. List all the foods and drinks and eateries that you know genuinely do bring you comfort on some level when you engage with them. These are what you will draw on. When eating out, know what you're going to allow yourself to eat in advance so you have room for manoeuvre, but not free rein. For the foods and drinks you buy in to eat at home, pre-buy these so they are there for you if you want

them, but – most importantly – set 'healthy' parameters for yourself about what your 'one-sitting limit' is for each of these items so you can eat them when you want to, but *not* go over the top.

3. Decide and act on one to three complementary therapies, practices or habits that will soothe you during this emotional time, or obtain professional counselling if necessary.

Now you've read about each type and the recommended action steps, it's time to write your unique list of action steps that you *know* will get you to your goal/s in a way that feels great to you.

My Unique Comfort-eating Plan

Write down your eating for comfort affirmation. Keep it with you and/or put it up somewhere you can see it every day. Example affirmation: 'It's OK to eat for comfort, but I know what'll feed and heal me best is attending to my heart.'

Now write your specific 'I am going to love this' action steps.

Now you have your plan, it's time to put it into action.

You can do this! This is your own personal recipe for creating a safe and loving space for yourself to feel to the degree that you feel comfortable with – without harming yourself in the process. As you go about creating this, ask yourself 'What would love do here?' and let this be your guide.

EATING FOR CONVENIENCE, LIFESTYLE AND CIRCUMSTANCE 🍎

Most people have a time in their life where what they eat is dictated by lifestyle and/or circumstance. Whether it's having to share a house or kitchen with someone who does the catering, or having to eat according to a tight budget, or eating on the road a lot, life has a way of giving us lots of different experiences, some of which often feel outside of our control.

If you are in a situation right now where, even though you'd love to pursue one of the other Possibilities, it's a case of 'needs must' coming first, this is for you. Within this final Possibility we're going to look at how you can turn what might feel like a burden into something that gets to work for you and something that you can even feel really good about.

Ready to achieve the so-called impossible?

Eating for convenience, lifestyle and circumstance is for you if:

- You're in a situation that you wouldn't call ideal

- You're limited to a budget and need to find a way to eat within your means

- Your living situation is currently in some state of disarray

- You don't have time to prepare freshly made meals

- You're not at home a lot of the time and have to eat on the road.

The Eater Types that you could run with or integrate for experiencing improved convenience, lifestyle and circumstance:

- **The Functional Eater** – will enable you to feel satiated on much less than you might be used to, as its needs are minimal and pretty straightforward.

- **The Sensual Eater** – will show you how to bring luxury into your diet in just the right amount and in clever ways you might not have thought about.

- **The Intellectual Eater** – will help you get really clear on what's what and what all your different options are.

- **The Focused Eater** – will give you set parameters to work to so that you never feel as if you are adding fuel to an already compromising situation.

- **The Experimental Eater** – will give you ideas for how to do things differently, whether it be trying a new shop or supplier, eating differently to feel greater pleasure, or trying different foods to get better results.

- **The Social Eater** – will encourage you to allow others to help and support you and for there to be more love and sharing in your life. This sense of community will pay huge dividends in your life.

Using Your Dominant Type in a Way That Works

Get Clear

Get clear on your goal and write it down – make it a SMART goal, that is: Specific, Measurable, Achievable, Realistic and Timely. Also, imagine how you will look and feel when you get there, and state it in the present tense as if it has already happened:

It is now 31st October 2012 and even though I am still living at home with my parents, I have found a way to socialize with them and be with them that actually feels progressive! Previously I was spending a lot of time (and money) eating takeaways on the way home from work, but after I lost my job and had to move in with them, everything had to change. At first I got sucked into their ways of doing things, living off meat and potatoes and

*drinking wine every night, but by working with my Type/s I have
come to create a way of eating that allows me to eat healthfully,
still feel decadent and treated and stay within my very limited
budget while I spend my days proactively looking for a new
place to work. I'm so glad that I took this approach, as I now see
that if I can make good of this situation then I can probably do
just about anything! I am grateful.*

Put It Up

Put your SMART goal somewhere you can see it every day,
multiple times per day. Consider making more than one copy
so that you can carry one in your wallet or purse.

Visualize It

See yourself – inside and out – feeling really good about your
circumstances even if they feel less than ideal. Feel how good it
feels to know that with every positive action you take, whether
it be with your diet or with any other lifestyle choice, you are
taking yourself another step closer to getting what you want.
Allow yourself to enjoy this Possibility and know that with every
step you take you *will* get where you want to be.

Commit to It

Commit to giving yourself this Possibility – in a way that works
for you. You are as entitled to be happy, fulfilled and joyful as
the next person, but to experience and have that you need
to make choices that allow you to have that. Remember, it all
starts (and ends) with you.

Action Steps

What follows are three powerful action steps per Eater Type
that will help you to create the most enjoyable and doable
eating plan for you according to your current circumstances.

If your current eating style is a combination of more than one Type, simply read the action steps for each Type and decide which action steps are going to work best for you. If you'd like to integrate action steps from other Types in order to try on a new Eater Type profile to create your specific eating for convenience, lifestyle and circumstance plan/guidelines, that's absolutely fine. However, do be clear that your main consideration is to be 'realistic', taking into account what you know about yourself, what resonates for you when you read about each Type, and what you have enjoyed and made work for you in relation to your lifestyle/circumstances so far.

Get a pen and paper to finalize your unique list of action steps. There is a Menu Plan template at the back of this book, or you can also download it for free (together with a special action steps sheet) at ERFYPTBonuses.com, to make the process super-easy and fun.

The Functional Eater

You need a convenience, lifestyle and circumstance plan that is quick and easy to follow and that involves minimum fuss, tastes delicious and helps you to reach your convenience, lifestyle and circumstance goals simply and easily.

Your Three Best-fit Action Steps

1. List all the foods you want to eat, that are a fit for your particular lifestyle/circumstance criteria, and where to get them (ideally pre-made) that will make this really easy for you. Next, list the mail order companies, local takeaways and other super-easy-to-use services that will give you exactly what you want with minimal input on your part.

2. Create or find a menu plan that is quick, easy and delicious to follow, that incorporates these pre-made foods and drinks wherever possible, and includes other meals that

you can quickly pull together yourself (in 10 minutes or less) that will be a perfect fit for your preferences/ situation.

3. Make three copies of your plan: one for your kitchen, one for your bedroom, one for your wallet or purse. Make sure you stick to it.

The Sensual Eater

You need a convenience, lifestyle and circumstance plan that satisfies all your senses, is just as pleasurable as your usual menu to eat (if not more so) and enables you to reach your convenience, lifestyle and circumstance goals deliciously and decadently.

Your Three Best-fit Action Steps

1. Buy or obtain some new chinaware, glassware or anything for your kitchen that delights and inspires you and celebrates you, regardless of your current circumstances.

2. Create or find a menu plan that excites you, where everything on your menu feels like a 10/10 for you, including foods and drinks that you consider treats or long-time favourites *and* that will be a perfect fit for your current preferences/situation.

3. Find sensual ways to reward and indulge yourself that are non-edible and also take into account your current preferences/situation. Think outside the box to get what you *really* want!

The Intellectual Eater

You need a convenience, lifestyle and circumstance plan that makes complete sense to you, with no questions left unanswered and that 'adds up' in your head to help you matter-of-factly reach your convenience, lifestyle and circumstance goals.

Your Three Best-fit Action Steps

1. List all the different criteria you need to take into account when creating your plan.

2. Create or find a menu plan that accommodates all of these criteria and also pleases you nutritionally, so you are truly happy about what you're eating.

3. Set a juicy 'turn this situation around' goal that feels realistic and achievable, together with a weekly action plan and chart where you can keep track of your progress and move towards what you really want instead.

The Emotional Eater

You need a convenience, lifestyle and circumstance plan that allows you to continue to use food in a way that nurtures you while using foods that enable you to conveniently adapt to your current lifestyle and circumstances.

Your Three Best-fit Action Steps

1. List 10 different non-edible treats that you know will 'fill you up' emotionally. Reach for these instead of food whenever possible. Make sure you give yourself what you really want and need.

2. Create or find a menu plan that honours the realities of whatever situation you are in, and nurtures you as much as possible – on every level.

3. Ask someone to support you in moving through your situation to create one that is fully supportive of what you want for yourself and who you want to be. In addition to this, or if you can't find such a person, spend a minimum

of 15 minutes daily writing in a journal, processing your feelings about your situation and planning how you are going to change things to get what you want instead.

The Focused Eater

You need a convenience, lifestyle and circumstance plan that is to-the-point, easy to follow, that is clearly going to work and enables you to reach your convenience, lifestyle and circumstance goals efficiently and enjoyably.

Your Three Best-fit Action Steps

1. Get really clear on where you're at right now and where you want to be. Create a game plan for turning things around.

2. Create or find a menu plan that accommodates the reality of your current situation while proactively supporting the pursuit and realization of the results you seek.

3. Invest in whatever tools, support or equipment you need to help you to change your situation successfully.

The Intuitive Eater

You need a convenience, lifestyle and circumstance plan that feels a great fit for you, allows you some flexibility depending on your hunger levels, and enables you to reach your convenience, lifestyle and circumstance goals sensitively.

Your Three Best-fit Action Steps

1. Make a list of foods that fit the following three criteria: the ones that your body is asking for right now, the ones that you know your body thrives on the most, the ones that fit within the confines of your current reality.

2. Create or find a menu plan that comprises these foods and that will also allow you to move beyond your current situation.

3. Pay close attention to your feelings during this time and look after yourself in the best ways possible with what you can do. Your priorities are to honour your whole self during this transition so that you do not spiral into emotional eating.

The Conscious Eater

You need a convenience, lifestyle and circumstance plan that satisfies your soul, is a perfect fit for your highest philosophy, and enables you to reach your convenience, lifestyle and circumstance goals easily and peacefully.

Your Three Best-fit Action Steps

1. Get really clear on where you're at right now and where you want to be. Create a nurturing and heart-led game plan for turning things around.

2. Create or find a menu plan that accommodates the reality of your current situation and comprises the foods that serve you best and play into your personal food philosophy.

3. Invest in whatever tools, support or equipment you need to help you change your situation as soon as possible to the way you want it to be.

The Experimental Eater

You need a convenience, lifestyle and circumstance plan that is as varied as you love things to be, introduces you to new and exciting foods, and allows you to reach your convenience, lifestyle and circumstance goals creatively and enthusiastically.

Your Three Best-fit Action Steps

1. Whatever situation you are in, think of all the ways you could 'get around' it and create the food experiences that you want for yourself, such as working at a restaurant, staying with friends, applying to be a food-taster.

2. Create or find a menu plan that still feels as exciting as ever to you, and that's realistic and achievable depending on what approach to your situation you decide to take.

3. Decide and act on creatively moving beyond any confines that may currently be constructing your life and work the plan to set you free.

The Confused Eater

You need a convenience, lifestyle and circumstance plan that makes total sense to you, raises no questions whatsoever, and that enables you to reach your convenience, lifestyle and circumstance goals confidently and purposefully.

Your Three Best-fit Action Steps

1. Get really clear on where you're at right now and where you want to be. Make the commitment and plan to move to that future place as soon as possible.

2. Create or find a menu plan that accommodates the reality of your current situation and comprises the foods that will best support you physically, emotionally and intellectually at this time.

3. Invest in whatever tools, support or equipment you need to help you change your situation as soon as possible to the way you want it to be.

The Social Eater

You need a convenience, lifestyle and circumstance plan that is fun and flexible to follow, that allows you to socialize as much as you've always done, and that enables you to reach your convenience, lifestyle and circumstance goals joyfully and playfully.

Your Three Best-fit Action Steps

1. Make a list of all the places or social gatherings you can eat at that are a fit for your current personal considerations.

2. Create a menu plan that incorporates these places, the meals you will eat while there as well as the everyday-at-home foods you like to eat, so you can feel prepared that all of your needs will be met, no matter where you may be.

3. Utilize your many connections to help you move beyond your current circumstances and into the reality you really want to be in.

Now you've read about each type and the recommended action steps, it's time to write your unique list of action steps that you *know* will get you to your goal/s in a way that feels great to you.

My Unique Convenience, Lifestyle and Circumstance Eating Plan

Write down your eating for convenience, lifestyle and circumstance affirmation. Keep it with you and/or put it up somewhere you can see it every day. Example affirmation: 'No matter what situation I am in, I can turn it around, create what I want and thoroughly enjoy the process.'

Now write down your specific 'I am going to love this' action steps.

Now you have your plan, it's time to put it into action.

You can do this! This is your own personal recipe for creating what you want in this particular chapter of your life. Know that as you get on your own side and move forward with the mindset that there is a way to have what you want, new ideas and approaches will open themselves up to you. Life is yours for the creating.

CHAPTER 5
What's Your Most Delicious Recipe?

Now that you know what your natural/default Eater Type profile is, the new one you want to move forward with, *and* the Possibility you are pursuing, it's time to bring it all together.

This is the time to make sure that the 'recipe for success' that you have come up with is indeed the right one for you – in fact, you need to love it so much that you would call it your most delicious recipe.

Over the next few pages you'll find some questions that will help you create your own unique delicious recipe – it's this that you'll move forward with and that will effectively help you reach your goal/s.

Note: if you have chosen more than one Possibility, amalgamate your answers within each question rather than running through the whole set of questions again for each one.

This is the final frontier, so make it count!

1. What is the Possibility you have chosen to pursue and why?

2. In relation to your chosen Possibility, what *specifically* do you want to be true for you, so that you can know you have succeeded?

3. How will your life be different as a result of getting what you want? (The more thought you can put into this answer, the more compelled you will be to make it happen.)

4. What Eater Type profile have you chosen to get you there and why? (Write your reasons down for each Type, so each one is validated.)

Deliciousness Test

For you to know that you have selected the right recipe for you, you must be able to say 'Yes' to each of the following statements. If one or more of the answers is a 'No,' then you need to go back to the relevant section/s of the book and select again as appropriate until you have all yeses. This is very important, because if you're not totally on board with what you've come up with then you'll find ways or reasons not to do what you've set out to do.

*   I am excited by the Possibility I have chosen to pursue.

*   I am really clear on why I want what I want.

*   I have personalized my Possibility so that the goals within it are perfect for me and what I want to create in my life.

*   I feel confident that the Eater Type profile I have chosen for myself is the right one and will get me where I want to go.

*   I am excited to start living with the Eater Type profile that I have come up with.

*   I have a good understanding of each of the Eater Types I have selected and know how to move forward with them.

*   If I should stumble along the way I will secure support for myself from those I love or a professional who can help me where I need help.

- I am fully committed to myself, my goals and the delicious recipe I have come up with for myself and can't wait to get started!

All done?

You will know you have got your most delicious recipe when you are smiling from ear to ear. It's that simple.

Once you're at this point, there are just a few more things I'd like to share with you before you get on your way. I'd like now to officially welcome you to the threshold to a whole new world, and show you how to pull together the final all-important steps you need to take to get you there.

CHAPTER 6
A Whole New World

There's no doubt about it: the process you have just learned can and will change your life – and not just once, but for the rest of your life.

Once you have truly grasped that the identity you take on and the way you nourish yourself together create your physical and physiological reality, quite literally a whole new world is opened up to you.

And within this new world lies not one, but *multiple* possible realities. Yes, we're talking about The 10 Possibilities you've already been introduced to, but, should you choose to go deeper, the lessons you will learn and the experiences you will have via your experiments and adventures with food and identity will introduce you to even more 'magical' possibilities for your body, life and your personal health and happiness *which will absolutely blow you away*.

If you want to learn more about this, you can read my own story about how I went from junk-food eater and butcher-shop worker to international raw food coach, teacher and trainer at www.ERFYPT.com. As I'm sure you can appreciate, the two identities I have operated from couldn't be more different – and the body and life I created with both were also at opposite ends of the spectrum – i.e. humdrum versus spectacular. No coincidence, I can assure you.

Therefore, the biggest gift I can give to you via our time together here is not simply to help you discover what type of eater you are and to help you create a whole new experience for yourself – although those are both fantastic tools to know about and utilize for sure, but actually to share with you that the closer attention you pay to who you are, what you want and how the food you put into your body shapes everything about you and your life, the more you will become master of your own domain – and when you have that, you have everything. Then, truly anything is possible.

In my work as a raw food coach and trainer, I would say that my key learnings over the past 19 years have been:

Be at Peace

The biggest service you can do for yourself and your body is to be at peace with whatever you are putting in to your body. This means that physically the food or drink nurtures and supports you, emotionally you feel happy and guilt-free about it, mentally you believe it to be good for you and that you are getting all the nutrition you need, and spiritually it facilitates more peace, clarity and connection. Rather interestingly, this may not (and usually does not) translate to following a specific prescribed food path that someone else has laid out for you (i.e. a dietary plan). It is for each of us to tune in to our most aware self on all those four levels and discover which foods and drinks suit us best as an individual at any given time. This way we get to be at peace with our choices, specifically because they are *our* choices, and they've come from a centred, intelligent, positive, awakened place within us.

Organic and Alive

The more 'alive' and organic foods that you put into your body (specifically: raw fresh fruits, leafy greens and vegetables, along with sprouted nuts, beans, seeds and grains), the more likely you are to find that place of peace and clarity, and very quickly too. This doesn't translate to eating *exclusively* fresh fruits, greens and vegetables however, although that can be massively transformational when consumed for a short period of time, but to use those as the basis for your diet, depending on which ones work best for you. Life force begets life force. It's as simple as that.

Keep It Clean

The cleaner you keep your diet – which means simply cooked or raw wholefoods and very little or no meat or dairy in the mix – the more connected and peaceful you will feel. This is because your body doesn't have to use its precious energy to 'deal' with less than wonderful things going into it. In this case, raw plant foods are once again superior and will both cleanse and rebuild, purifying you from the inside out. When this energy becomes available you'll find that suddenly you have much more energy to do much more exciting things with your life than eat!

Eat When You're Hungry

Eating when you're actually hungry is the key to peace, longevity, weight management and really enjoying food to the maximum. It is also your body's way of saying to you when it is ready to consume more food – a voice that usually doesn't get heard because most people do not let themselves experience true hunger. When you allow yourself to wait until you get hungry, a newfound respect and relationship with your body starts to blossom, and the realization that your body has never been out to get you hits you like a brick! It's great to know that you can trust your body and that it's been doing its best, despite less than optimum conditions. Just think what it can do when you actually work *with* it!

Know Who You Are

The ultimate key to eating joyfully and having a healthy and happy relationship with food is to know who you are and what you want, and to eat accordingly. This is the process I have shared with you, and it will free you up in myriad ways to help you become master of your own domain and to reinvent yourself and your life any time you want.

Sharing this Process with Others

Once you've benefited from this knowledge yourself, you'll likely want to share it with others. After all, who doesn't want to know more about themselves, especially when it comes to food?! People will love to find out what Eater Type they are, just as you have.

For this reason, I recommend that you start by asking your friends, family and work colleagues to take the 'What Type of Eater Are YOU?' quiz, then let them read about their Type/s themselves so they can really get a feel for what it's all about. They can do this via the book or online at www.ERFYPT.com. If they find the process interesting and want to know more then they'll need to work through the book from start to finish. This is important. None of the steps outlined in this book should be skipped, otherwise the process is incomplete and they won't know what they're doing or understand fully how and why the process works.

Sharing this process with others doesn't just benefit them, by the way. By knowing what Type/s your partner, best friend, children, etc. are, you'll find yourself much more understanding, accommodating and sympathetic towards their choices, plus you'll also be able to help them upgrade their diets and choices if they're open to it, because you'll know exactly how to go about it!

Taking Things to Another Level

For you and anyone else who wants to learn more or go further with this process, please refer to the Resources section on page 268, where there is information about the free bonus gifts available to you online.

One of the most important things I want to share with you through these gifts is the ERFYPT Pyramid of Evolution. This shows clearly what four types are foundational and to be evolved from, what three types are thinking/feeling – which is the next stage we move to – what two types are more spiritual/conscious (this is where we start making food choices from a less self-focused or one-dimensional perspective) and what one type sits at the top of the pyramid, harnessing all the other types into a place of mastery.

As you can tell, this is very powerful information – perfect for those who want to understand the inner workings of the process and the hierarchy of the types as referred to in Chapter 1. You can access this via the special download link given in the Resources section.

Pulling It All Together

We have covered a lot of ground during our work together – and much of it pretty big stuff! I want to congratulate you for choosing to focus on yourself and your own growth in this way. You should feel proud. By learning the ERFYPT process, you have enabled yourself to take control of your diet, body and life in a way that would not otherwise have been possible. And from that, many fantastic things can and will likely happen.

Now is the time to make sure that what you have learned gets implemented rather than forgotten. This information is far too precious to let go of – especially when you could be creating a much better body and life for yourself!

With this in mind, here are the action steps you need to take to move this work out of the book and into your world.

Step 1

Make sure you have completed all the exercises within this book and have transferred all the relevant information to your Eat Right For Your Personality Type Personal Success Blueprint on pages 257–58 (also available as a download – see page 268).

Step 2

Use the Menu Plan template on page 259 (also available as a download – see page 268) to map out your weekly schedule so you know what times you can shop, eat and prepare food to suit your own unique lifestyle.

Step 3

Use the ingredients listed on pages 253–55 together with the simple recipe ideas within the Eater Types section to complete your menu, making sure that everything you choose also aligns with the Possibility you have chosen for yourself. (This is super-important! Anyone can put together a menu, but your menu is effectively your route to success, so *everything* matters.) If you need extra help with this, refer to the ERFYPT.com website for some sample menu plans to guide and inspire you.

Step 4

Write a list of any actions you need to take, either directly from your Eater Type profile in Chapter 1 and/or that you have come up with independently. These might be new foods or ingredients to buy, investing in a new piece of kitchen equipment, detoxing your kitchen to make way for the new lifestyle you're creating, having a conversation with other members of your household so they know what you're doing and why you're doing it (and can support you or join you)… and more.

Step 5

There's only one thing left to do now – start living it!

Yes, the time has come to eat right for your personality type. And of course, I'm beyond fascinated to know who you were when you started reading the book, and now, out the other side, who you've decided to be.

If you'd like to share your journey with me and with others, then I'd love to hear from you via our special Facebook page. Simply visit www.ERFYPT.com to access it and let us know what Eater Type/s you were, what you've decided to be and what Possibility you're pursuing – and of course, how you're finding it and what you've achieved so far.

I can't wait to hear what you have to say. I'm wishing you all the very best for your amazing new life and everything that happens along the way. I'll see you there!

Great Foods For Healthy Eating

Generally speaking, these are great as part of a healthy diet for all types, depending on personal preference:

- fresh fruits
- vegetables
- leafy greens
- nuts
- seeds
- beans
- wholemeal/seeded bread
- rye bread
- sprouted bread
- wholegrain/basmati rice
- wholegrain/buckwheat/vegetable pasta
- rice cakes
- oat cakes
- no-sugar, no-additives muesli
- no-sugar, no-additives wholegrain cereal

- fresh fruit smoothies
- fresh green smoothies
- fresh fruit juices
- fresh vegetable juices
- fresh green juices
- kombucha
- wholegrain rolls, wraps or pittas with salad/avocado filling
- falafel
- jacket potatoes
- boiled potatoes
- fries alternative: boiled potatoes tossed in olive oil, apple cider vinegar and Celtic sea salt
- hummus
- vine wraps
- goat's cheese
- feta cheese
- mozzarella cheese
- cottage cheese
- boiled eggs
- sushi
- low-fat, no-additives vegetable curry
- egg noodle stir-fry with fresh veggies and soy sauce
- low-fat, no-additives soups
- couscous
- bean salads

- crudités with healthy low-fat, no-additives dips
- rice milk
- almond milk
- low-fat/non-dairy/organic yoghurts
- raw food snack bars
- raw ice-cream
- raw ice-cream sundaes
- raw food takeaways
- raw chocolate bars
- raw chocolate dipping sauce

Eat Right For Your Personality Type
Personal Success Blueprint

*'Choosing and creating a different reality for myself is easy.
When I get clear on what I want and who I need to be to get
there, I get to experience whatever my heart desires.'*

My default/original Eater Type profile is…

_____

_____

_____

Things I love about the way I currently eat/approach foods I
love and don't want to change…

_____

_____

_____

Things that I will no longer do when it comes to food/eating
because they stop me experiencing what I want…

_____

_____

_____

The Possibility I want to pursue and create for myself is…

_____

_____

The specific goal/s I am setting for myself in relation to the Possibility I am pursuing is/are...

_____

_____

_____

My new 'this will get me there' Eater Type profile that I'm going to move forward with is...

_____

_____

_____

The specific actions that I am going to take to embody this profile and reach my goals are...

1. _____

2. _____

3. _____

4. _____

5. _____

6. _____

7. _____

8. _____

9. _____

10. _____

The juicy reward I will give myself for reaching my goal/s is...

_____

_____

_____

MENU PLAN TEMPLATE

	MON	TUE	WED	THU	FRI	SAT	SUN
BREAKFAST							
LUNCH							
DINNER							
DRINKS							
SNACKS							

Frequently Asked Questions

Chapter 1: What Type of Eater Are You?

Q: What if my existing Eater Type profile is already perfect for me?
A: That's great if that's genuinely the case. My first suggestion is to complete all of the exercises just to make sure. If it's still the case, then that's fantastic – the only work you will have to do is simply choose the Possibility you want to pursue, design your menu plan and start experiencing the magic of conscious eating!

Chapter 2: So How's That Working For You?

Q: In my list of what I want to do more of and eradicate to feel happier, I have two answers conflicting with one another. I wrote that I want to eat out at swanky restaurants more often to make my Sensual/Social Eater happier, but I also want to save money because eating out and also buying high-quality foods is pretty harsh on my wallet. What do I do?
A: Great question! The answer is that there's almost always a way to make both things work even when they seem totally conflicting – you just have to look for it. In this case, I would recommend that you first decide on what your monthly food spend is, which will need to cover *all* food purchases whether they are for your home, when eating out

on the fly, and when dining out. You'll have to be rigorous about this or nothing will change, but don't be tight with yourself as it's clearly really important to you and you don't want to feel pinched – that would totally defeat the object and you won't get what you want.

Once you've done that, get clear on how that split needs to look so that it all works, and specifically that you have the money you need to eat out to the degree you want and where you want. Hopefully this works out financially for you; otherwise you'll need to find a rich partner to dine out with or earn more money! Either way, one way that you can economize, which will definitely make a difference, is to stop spending money on takeaways and weekday lunches that you could make at home. These 'here and there' costs can easily add up over the course of a month and therefore equate to a night out in a fancy restaurant. (For example, spending just £6 per day on lunch from a sandwich bar, which is a conservative amount anyway, would equal about £120 per month. If you brought your lunch from home you could easily cut that figure in half and enjoy it just as much, if not more, as you'd be using foods that you had picked yourself.) So, as you can see it can be done, you just need to take the time to figure out how this is going to look so you can get what you want – and you don't need me to tell you that every second will be time well spent.

Chapter 3: Everything Changes Right Here

Q: I'm fascinated by the concept of seeing food as energy, no matter what food group it might fall into; it's really made me think. My question is, how can I start to 'read' the energy of foods to know which ones are good for me and which aren't?

A: I love this question! Reading the energy of different foods and drinks is actually easier than you might think, and some of this you will likely already know. For example, if you think about it you're probably aware that the energy of bread is calming and mildly sedating. That is, when you eat it your energy goes down a little and you don't feel very rock and roll! When you think about chocolate, you probably know only too well that its energy is comforting and 'dreamy' – when eating it you can feel transported to a different, more welcoming place. These are just two simple examples, but I know you can think of many more. By starting with the most common ones and really thinking about how they make you feel when you eat/drink them – or tuning in to your body the next time you do – you'll soon find that you have the ability to 'read' all manner of other foods and drinks, too – even without consuming them! This is a gift that I believe all of us can uncover, and there's no doubt that cleaning up your diet and your body will be the biggest help of all in enabling you to tune in in this remarkable and invaluable way. Uncovering and using this gift really does set you on the path to food- and self-mastery.

Chapter 4: The Plate of Possibilities

Q: I want to experience all of The 10 Possibilities! Where do I start?
A: Start with where you are today and what's most important to you right now at this particular point in your life. Also, think logically: if you feel you need to have realized one Possibility before another is possible, then you'll need to pursue that one first – so you'll definitely need to apply common sense as well. Don't worry – you have plenty of time to master and enjoy them all if that's what you want!

Chapter 5: What's Your Most Delicious Recipe?

Q: How do I choose a new Eater Type profile without becoming confused or overwhelmed?
A: If you're feeling overwhelmed it's likely to be because you're trying to take too much on. This might be because you're entertaining the idea of pursuing more than one Possibility. If this is the case, then whittle it down to just one. If you're simply overwhelmed at the thought of understanding the 10 different Eater Types, stop, take a deep breath, read the simple summaries of each Type at the start of each one in Chapter 1 and take it from there. The Types are so different to one another it shouldn't take too much to choose the right one/s for you. You'll just know which one/s feel right.

Q: What do I do when I reach my goals?

A: First, celebrate and reward yourself – that's very important (although some think that reaching the goal is reward enough, I personally don't!!). Second, quickly run yourself through the exercises in the first two chapters to see if anything needs tweaking and then, re-read through the 10 different Possibilities and choose yourself another. Make it as refined, exciting or challenging as you desire. Then, off you go again!

Menu Planning

Q: How do I eat more healthily and indulge my 'naughty' side?

A: There are plenty of foods that feel decadent, luxurious and/or naughty that are really good for you. Some examples are: apricots, avocado, bananas, blackberries, blueberries, cherimoya (custard apple), cherries, fresh dates, dragon fruit, durian, figs, grapes, guava, jackfruit, kumquats, lychees, mango, mangosteen, melon, mulberries, nectarines, olives, papayas, passion fruit, peaches, persimmon, physallis, pineapple, plums, pomegranates, raspberries, star fruit, strawberries, tamarind, watermelon; asparagus, beetroot, fresh herbs; almonds, Brazil nuts, cashews, coconut (old and young), hazelnuts, macadamia nuts, peanuts, pecans, pine nuts, pistachio nuts; dried apple rings, dried apricots, dried cherries, dried cranberries, dried figs, goji berries, dried mango, dried mulberries, dried papaya, dried peach, dried pineapple, prunes; almond oil, avocado oil, olive oil, sesame oil; raw chocolate powder, raw chocolate bars; vanilla essence, vanilla pods.

These are obviously just ingredients, but of course there is no end to what you can create with them! And then there are store-bought pre-prepared items that cater to the more discerning palate, everything from gourmet breads with wholesome ingredients to rich, additive-free, flavourful soups, or something more exotic – it all depends on what you fancy!

Whatever your personal tastes and definition of 'naughty', just know that there are plenty of options for you and you don't have to trade health for happiness *at all*.

One of my personal favourite things to make that feels decadent, celebratory *and* is super-healthy all at once, are 'mocktails' using fresh fruit juice (which I juice myself), sparkling water and anything else that takes my fancy and will give it that *je ne sais quoi* factor. I love serving these in tall, elegant wine glasses and creating new recipes that get better every time.

Truly, when you set the intention to 'have it all' – whatever that looks like for you – you will find a way to create it that works for you, because infinite possibilities exist. You just have to name it and claim it for yourself.

Q: My partner is the complete opposite to me in eating habits and, to be honest, it can be very stressful. I often end up compromising just so he is happy – but then I'm not. How can we make it work?
A: Ah, I know this one well! When I first met my partner, I was a Functional/Intuitive/Focused Eater and he was a 100 per cent Sensual Eater. This meant that while I was trying to be quick, conscious and intentional around my food, he just wanted to eat whatever tasted good! In real life this translated as him being fussy about what he'd eat at home, wanting to dine out a lot (and I hardly ever ate out at that point) and he would 'overdo himself' (as my son liked to call it!) while I always stopped eating when I was full.

At first I really did wonder if we were going to be compatible for the long term, especially as food is my vocation and one of my passions and I'd spent years getting to where I wanted to be with it… but what ended up happening, and actually pretty quickly, was that we found some common ground that was great, although it did take a little tweaking on both sides.

For my part, I started trying new foods, expanding my horizons and appreciating him for his own version of foodie passion. I even started to look forward to eating out, as I could see how much pleasure it brought him and, eventually, me too. For his part, as he became inspired by my level of health, energy, consciousness around food and physique, he started paying much closer attention to what *he* was eating, cut out most of the junk and high-fat foods, joined the gym and lost over 14 lb in a few short weeks. He still remained a Sensual Eater (and is extremely proud of it!), but with the new element of Focused Eater in the mix, it meant that he stopped overeating and eating foods that weren't good for him, and his choice of restaurant and meals both in and out of the house evolved to a standard that made me really happy for both of us. So it *can* be done!

Through sharing this work with others, the best solution to this 'problem' has become very clear: first, both of you have to do this work and create specific goals for yourselves, and ideally also as a team. In doing this you'll find that you'll both automatically be wanting to eat more healthily, *and* both of you will be growing increasingly conscious around food, which can only ever be a good thing. Also, having individual and especially joint goals will make all the difference. As soon as you do this work you'll find that your two paths will start converging almost immediately; the only difference then between you may be around your different supporting Types – which may end up being quite fun and bring added interest. The dominant Type, meanwhile, will likely end up being the Focused Eater, which is really how it should be for anyone who is trying to get and stay aware around food. This process really does work, and not only for couples but also for children – try it!

Q: What if something I love about the way I eat now, and would ideally want to keep, is also the same thing that is stopping me from where I want to be?

A: This is a common quandary. This is where you'll have to choose between indulgence and results. If you choose the former, don't expect anything much to change (that is, unless you implement portion control, which could make enough of a difference – try it and see). If you want results, and especially if you want them fast, then just know that your results will come as thick and fast as the speed at which you let go of the thing/s that are holding you back.

Sharing Information

Q: *What's the best way to share this process with my friends and family?*

A: See page 248 for more specific guidelines about this, but, in summary you can either get them to take the What Type of Eater Are YOU? quiz, or work through the whole process as outlined in this book, just as you have done.

Q: *I'm a trained nutritionist and I'd love to use this process with my clients, as I can see how it would make all the difference to personalizing different eating plans and helping people stay with a particular eating programme. How can I use your methodology?*

A: I totally agree that this process would lend itself well to nutritionists as well as many other health-promoting professionals, which is why a training and licensing programme has been created. The training goes deeper into the content shared within this book and how to work with it with others, as you describe. To find out more, please visit www.ERFYPTTraining.com.

Resources

If you'd like to take your exploration and implementation of the ERFYPT system further, here are some resources to help you do just that.

Go to: www.ERFYPTBonuses.com to download your free ERFYPT kit containing:

1. The ERFYPT Pyramid of Evolution Chart

2. The 10 ERFYPT Recipes as featured in this book

3. The ERFYPT Ingredients List

4. A blank ERFYPT Menu Plan template for creating your own personalized menu

5. A fill-in-the-blanks ERFYPT Personal Success Blueprint poster.

To visit the main Eat Right For Your Personality Type website to read Karen's story, view sample menu plans and take the What Type of Eater Are YOU? quiz online, go to: www.ERFYPT.com

To learn more about training to become a certified ERFYPT teacher and/or using it in your own company or practice, go to: www.ERFYPTTraining.com